THE STORY OF CANCER
Volume 1

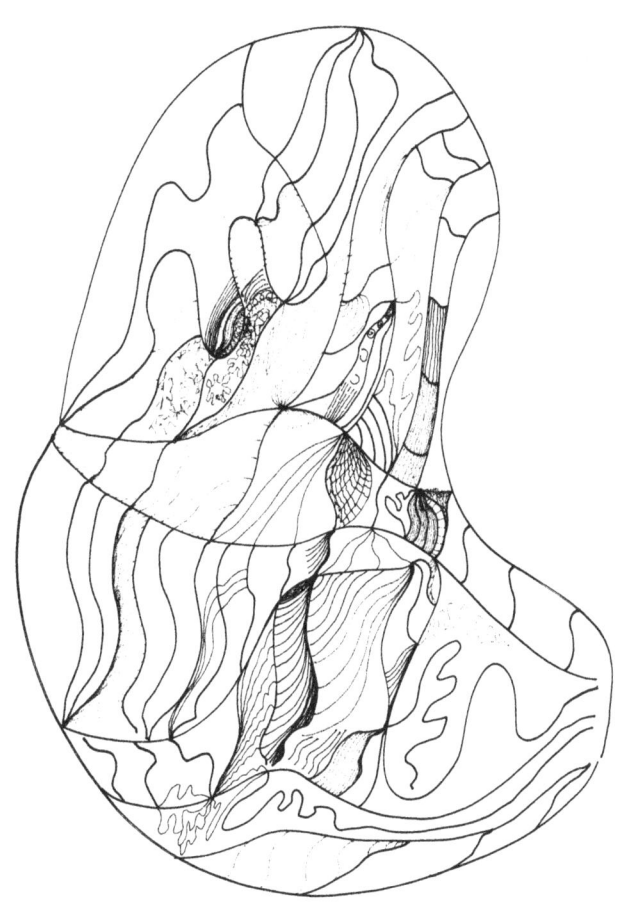

Camilia MacPherson, Ph.D., D.Th.
2016

INTRODUCTION

This is the Story of Cancer written in an unusual form. Automatic Drawings and Surreal Art are used to convey meaning. It is written in the style of Scholars' Art, a pre-calligraphy form of writing scholarly works dating as far back as 400 BC. It is one continuous document. The document begins with volume 1 and ends with volume 7. There are over 900 pages, each page consisting of several images. There are therefore several thousand images in this work.

This collection is not doodling emerging out of the subconscious as Automatic Drawings are often described.

The markings are quite sophisticated. The following diagram gives a glimpse of the complexity of this form of writing.

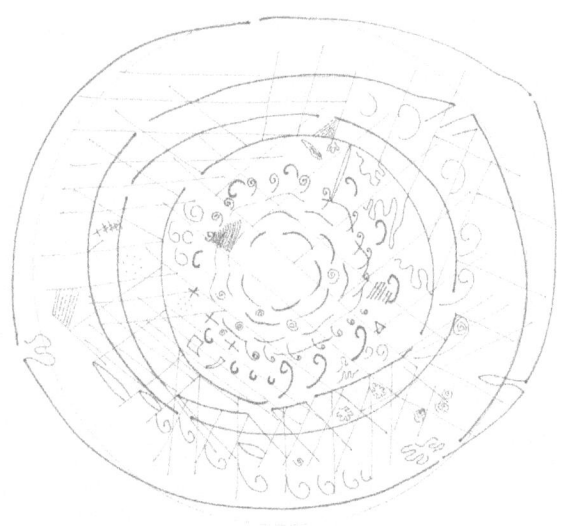

A scientific mind will naturally ask the question: Where are these images coming from? The question is quite complex since we are moving into the realm of the inexpressible. Inadequate explanations borrow from universal theologies. The Atman = Brahman formula meaning not equality but non-duality between the innermost Self and Brahman is encountered. The Trikaya also sheds some light. The Nirmanakaya emerges out of the Dharmakaya temporarily, enters into human space and participates within the human being as saving grace to help humanity. One can also say that the writer bypasses the 'waking state,' the 'dream state,' the 'dreamless sleep state,' enters into the state of Turiya and then returns to the conscious state retaining images derived from the fourth of the fourth. It is sometimes argued that there are four stages within the state of Turiya. There are many inadequate explanations for this phenomenon.

How does one read these images? Every page has to be looked at from every angle and varying depths. There is a surplus of meaning in every page. The logical scientific conscious mind is not sufficient in unlocking the meaning of these images. The intuitional and meditative aspects of the reader need to be awakened in order to grasp the full meaning of each image.

Several pages were written in colour and therefore lost some of its meaning. I chose black and white, rather than greyscale or colour since 99% of the drawings were in black and white. Unfortunately, I had to break up the one document into seven volumes due to the size required for uploading the file.

There is no top or bottom of the page. The line at the bottom of images come from the scanner. Lastly, before realizing the importance of this work, I had utilized paper and pens of a poor quality.

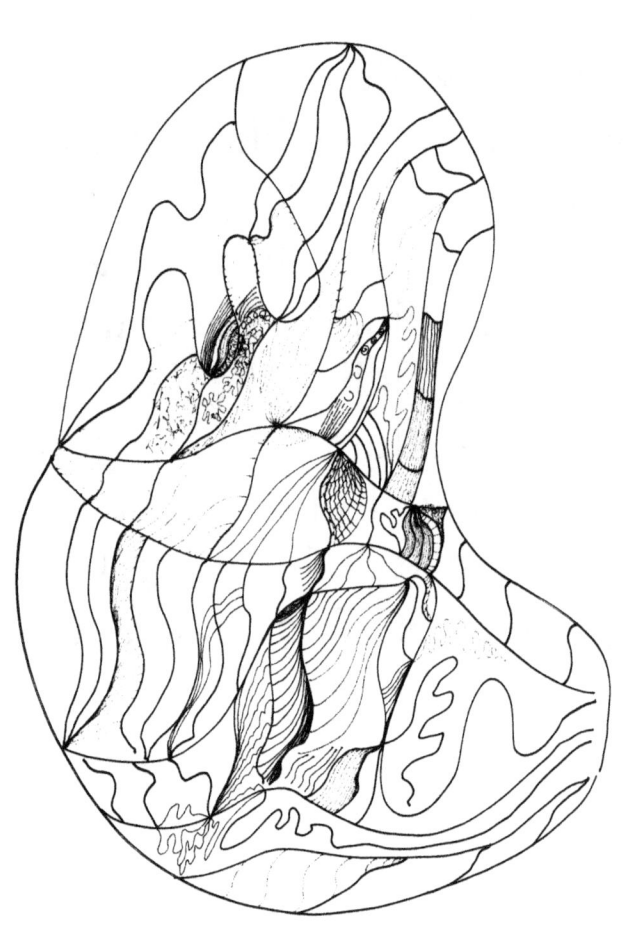

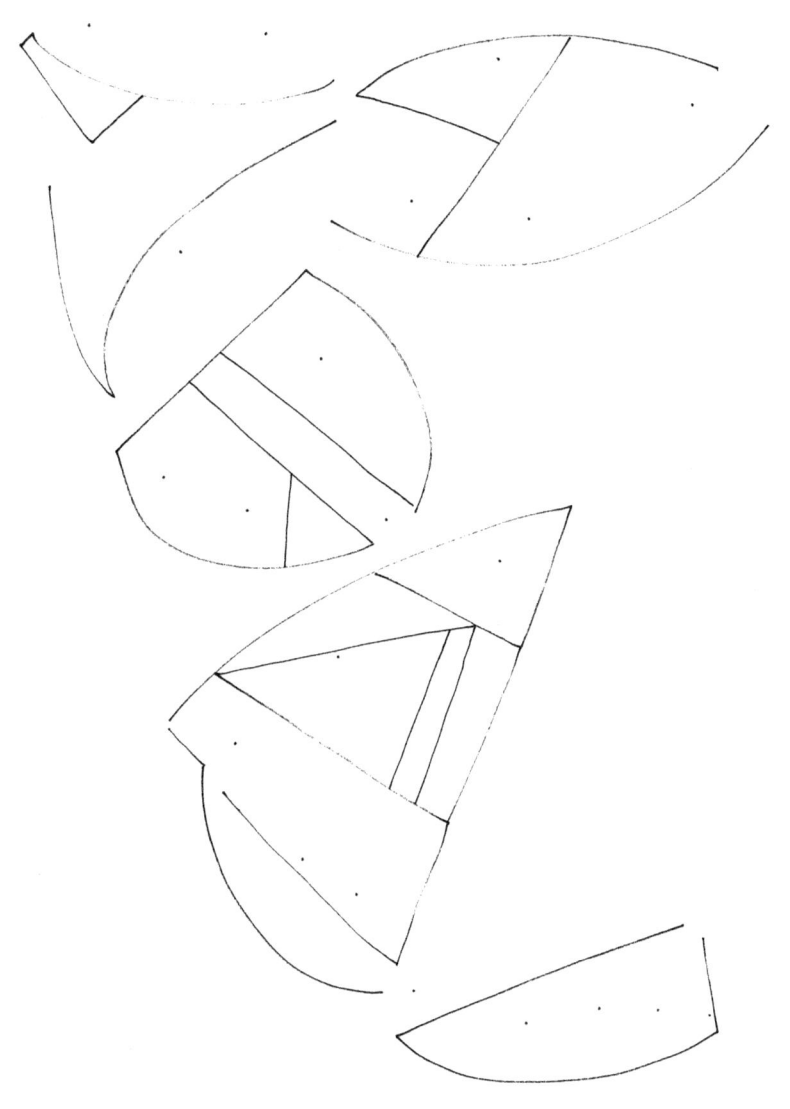

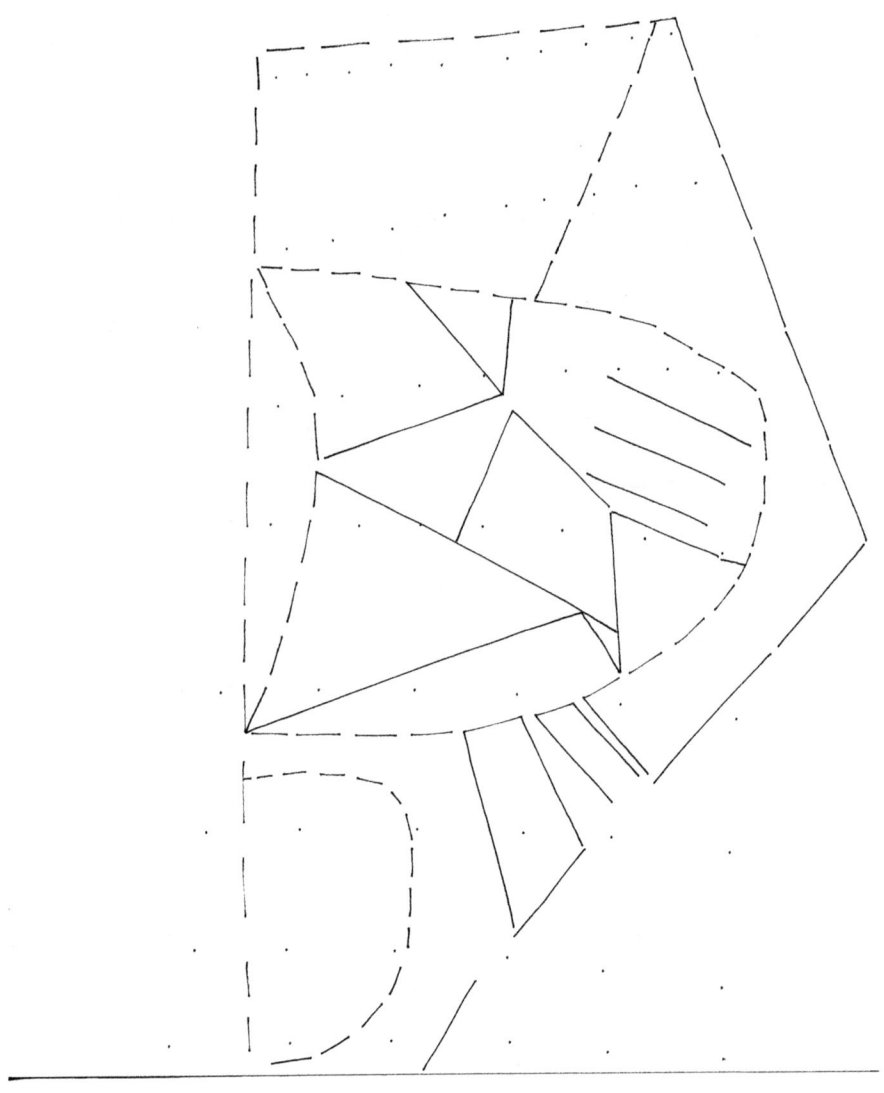

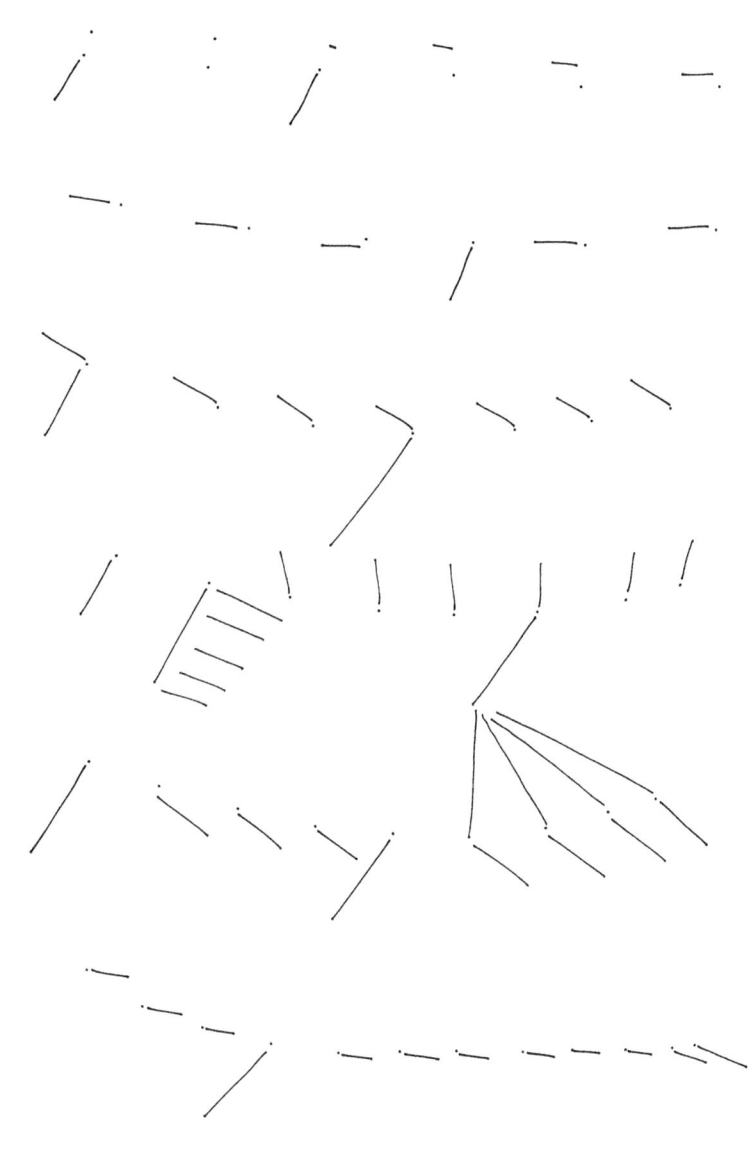

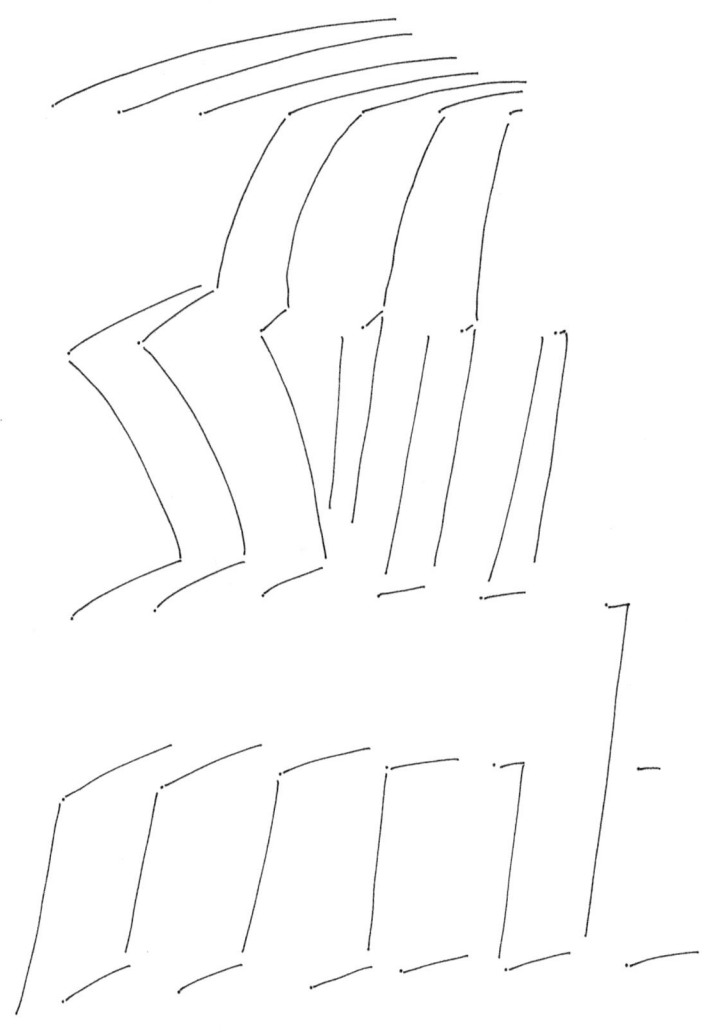

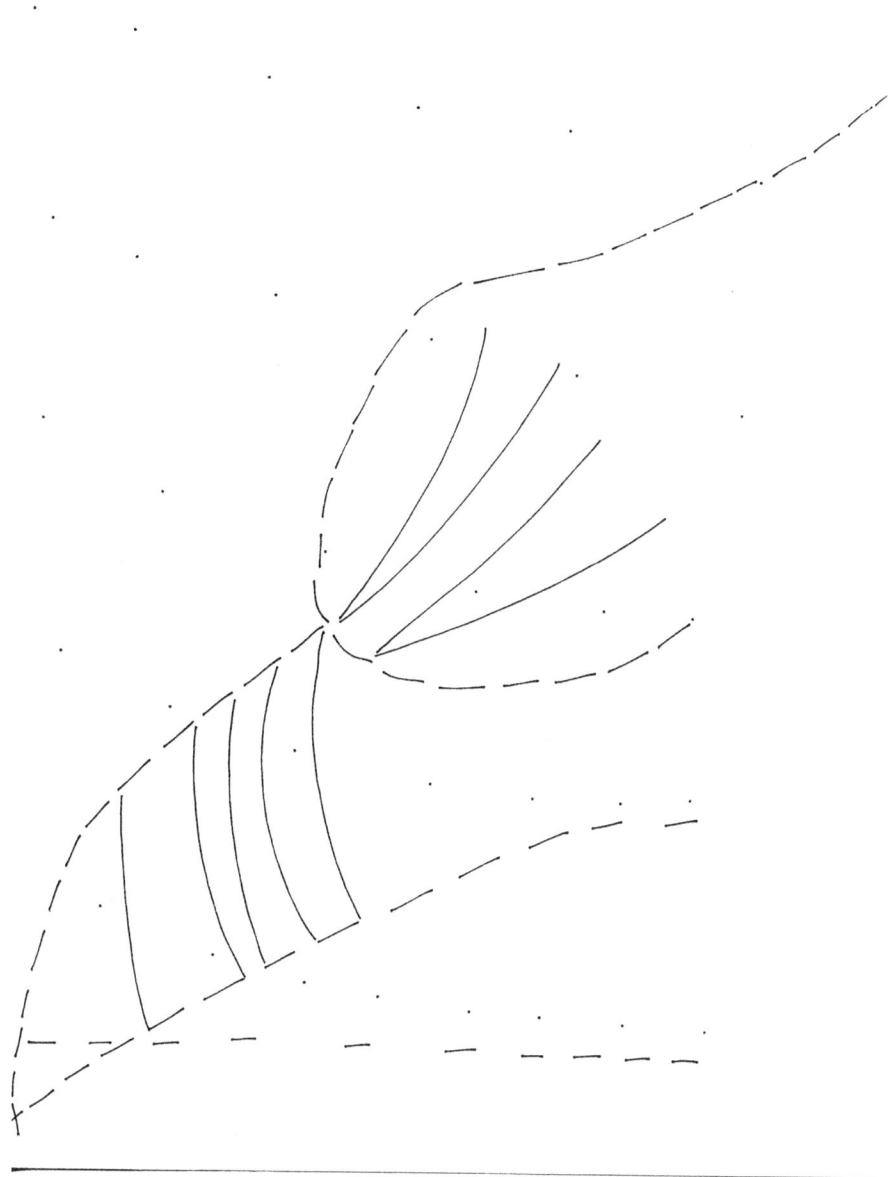

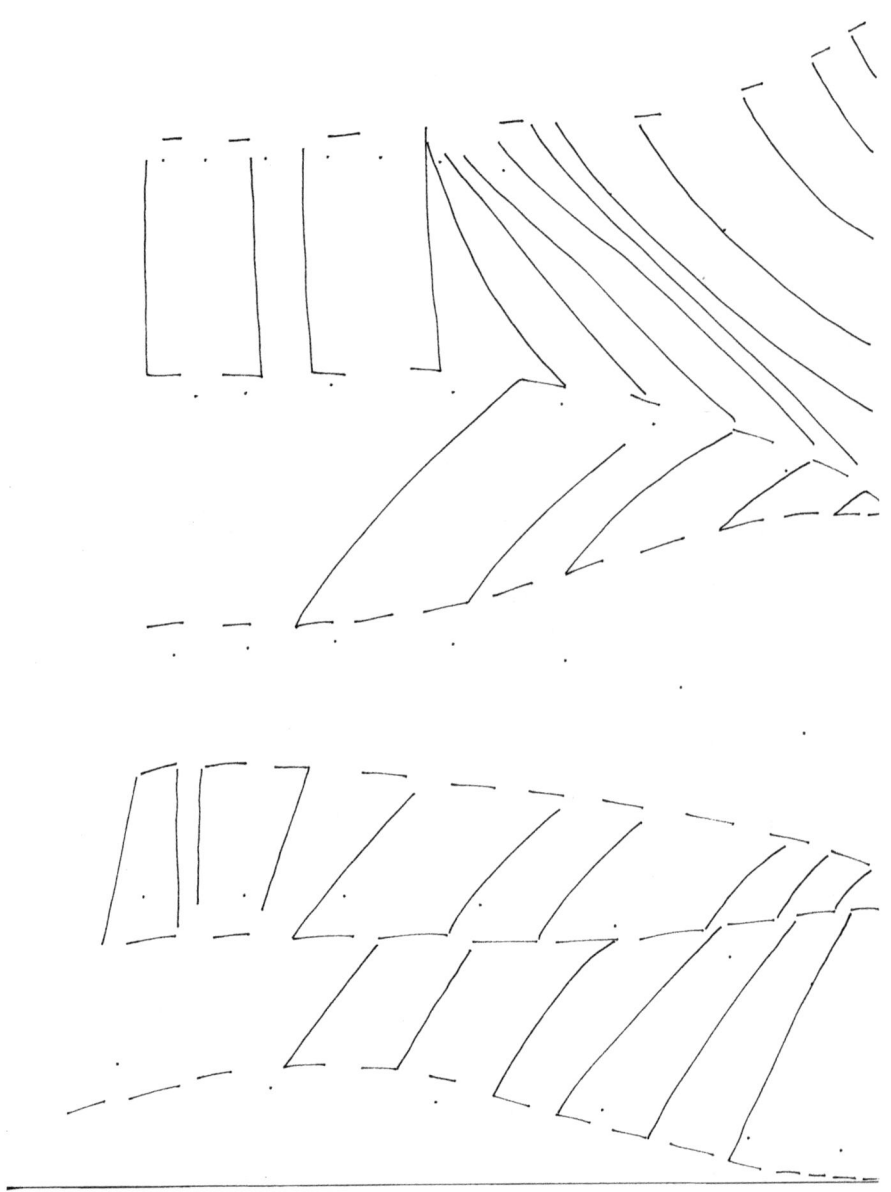

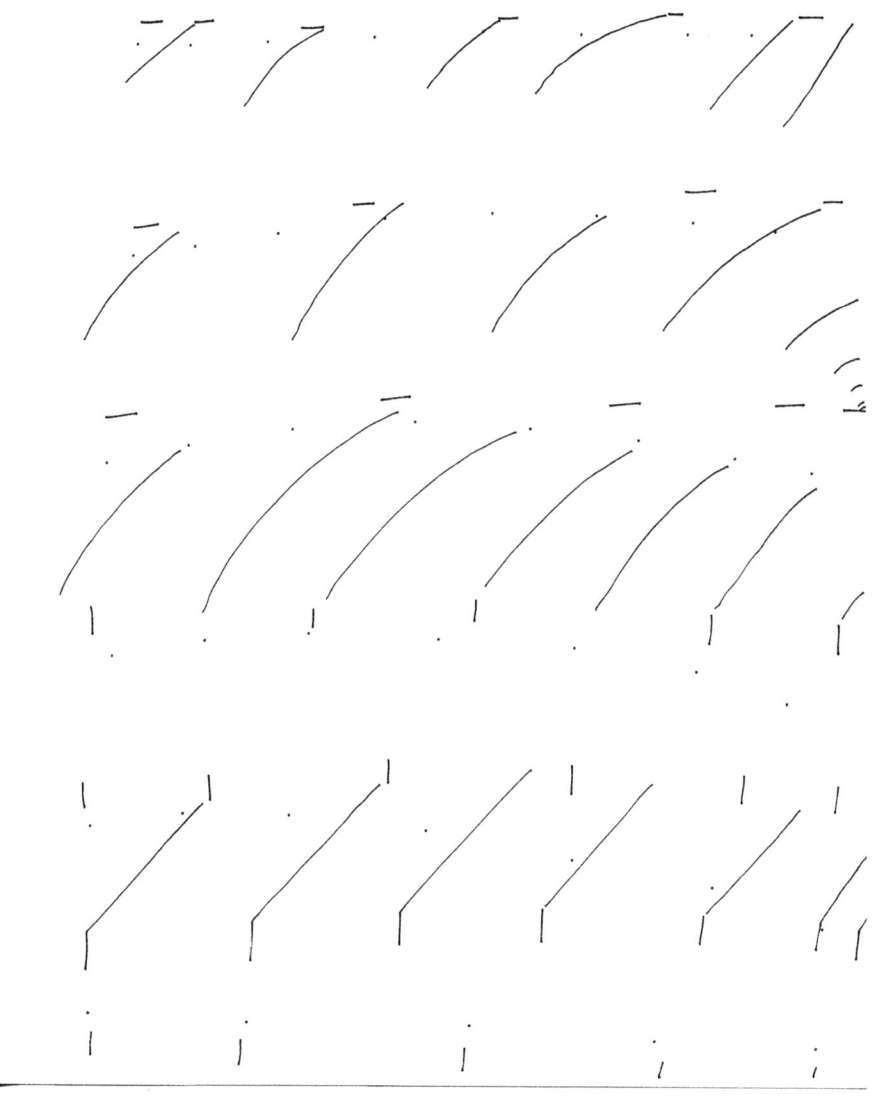

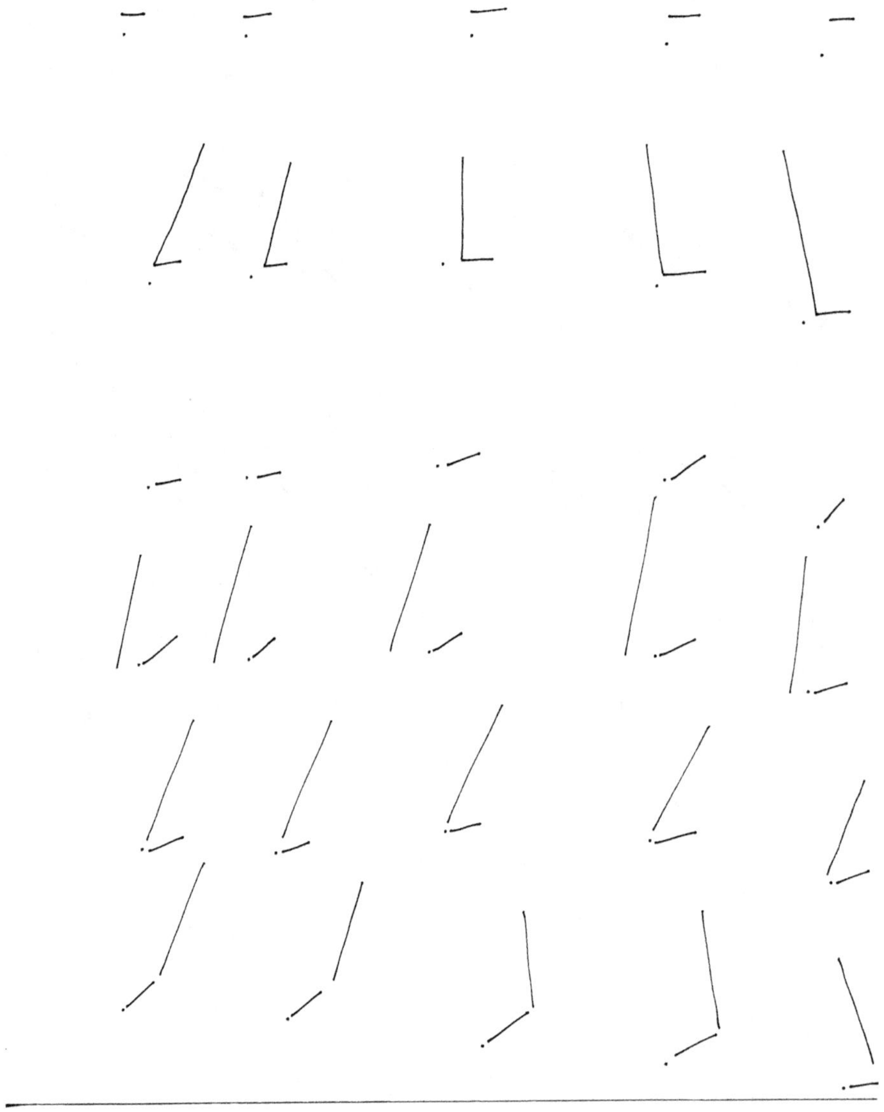

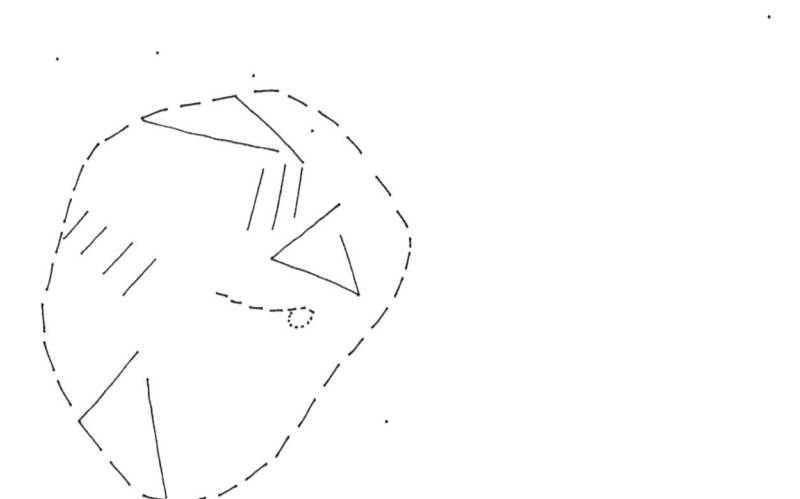

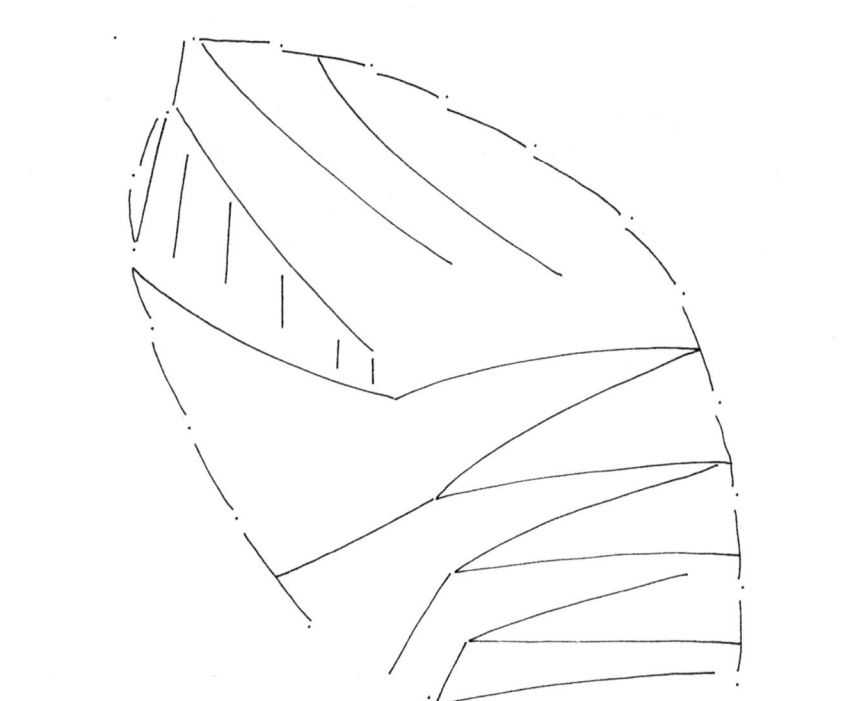

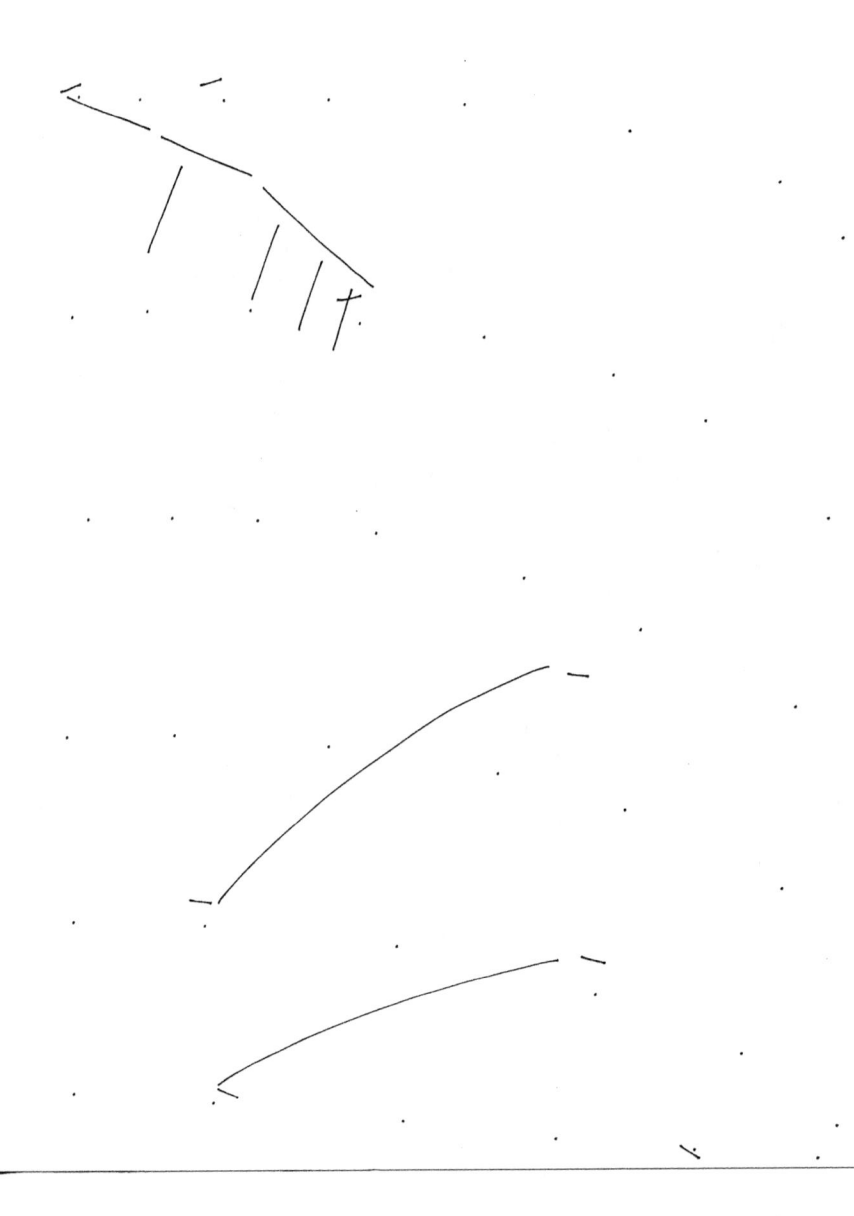

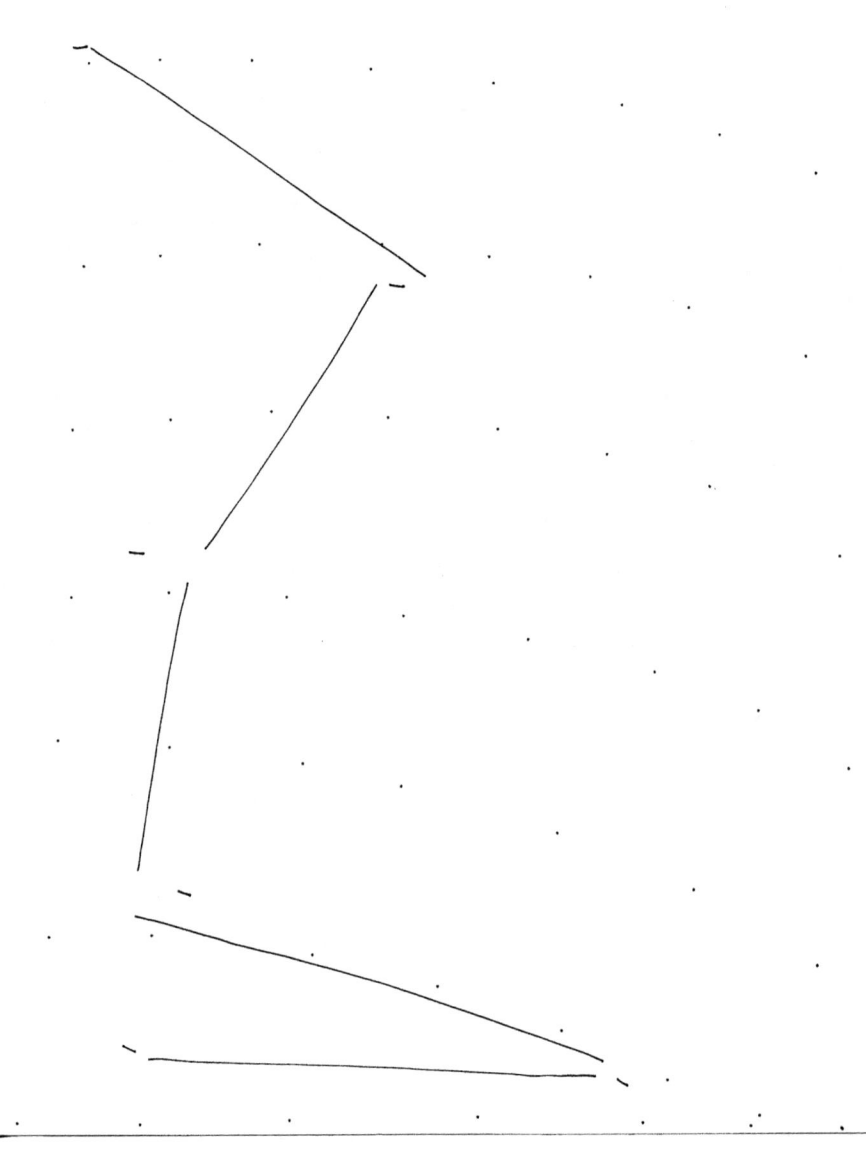

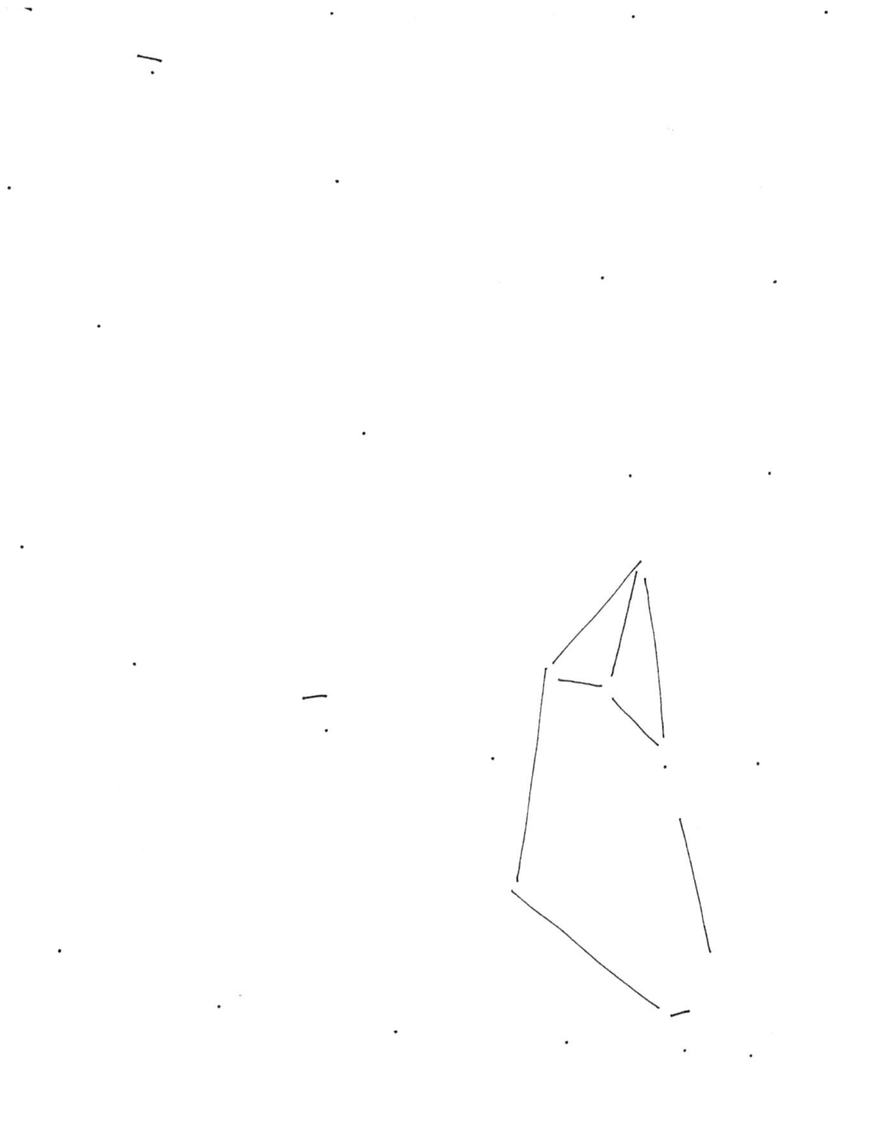

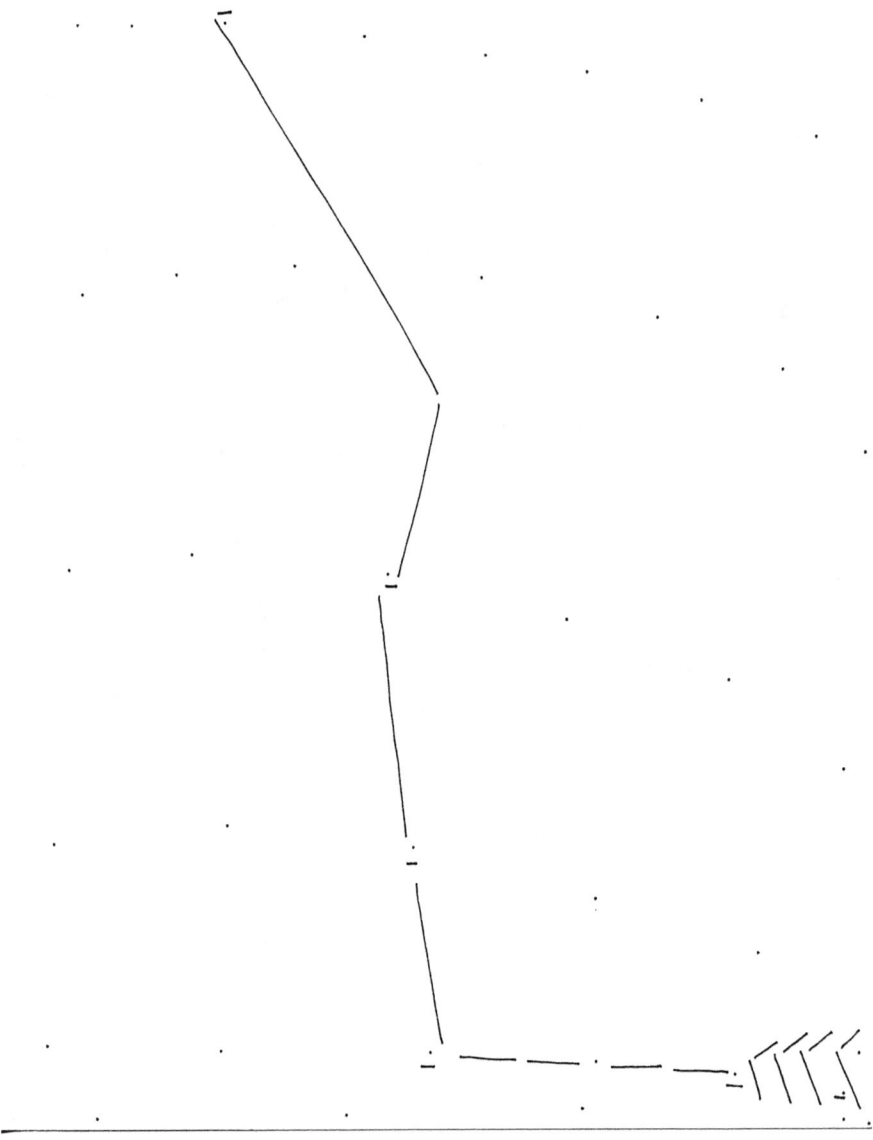

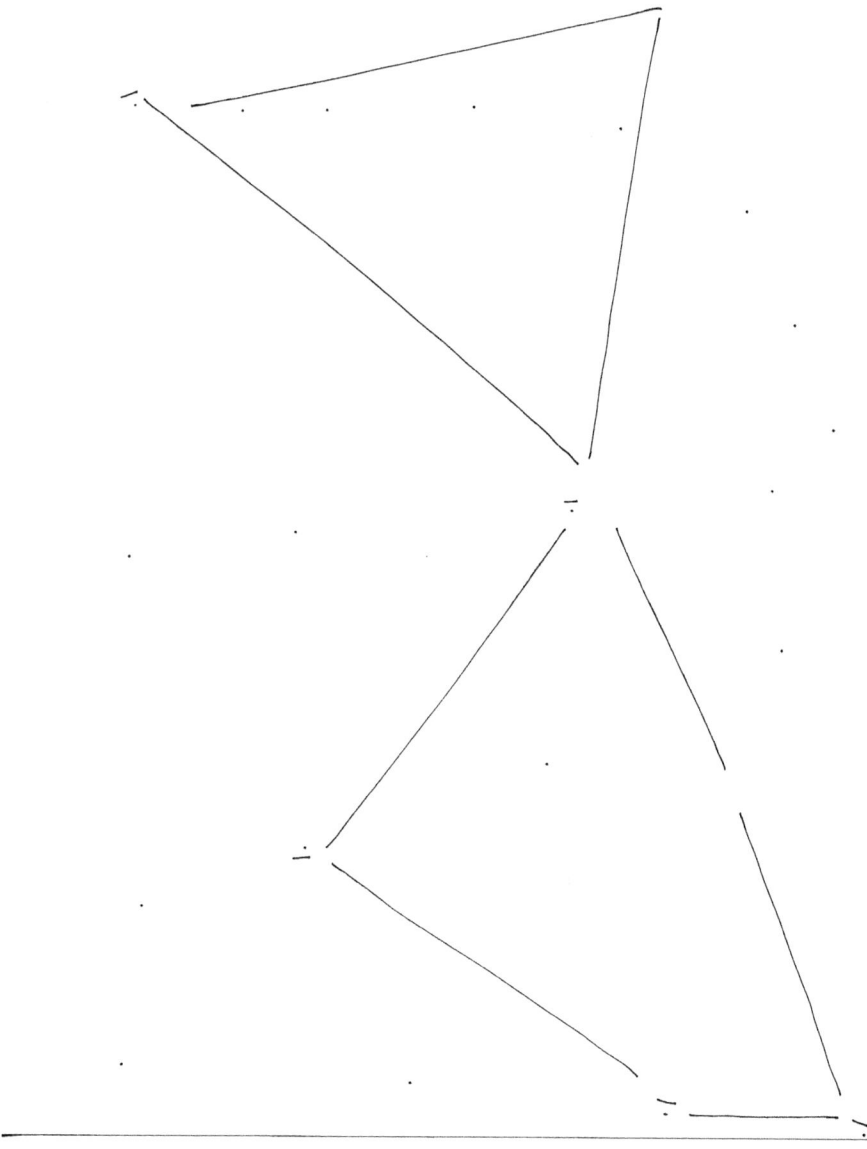

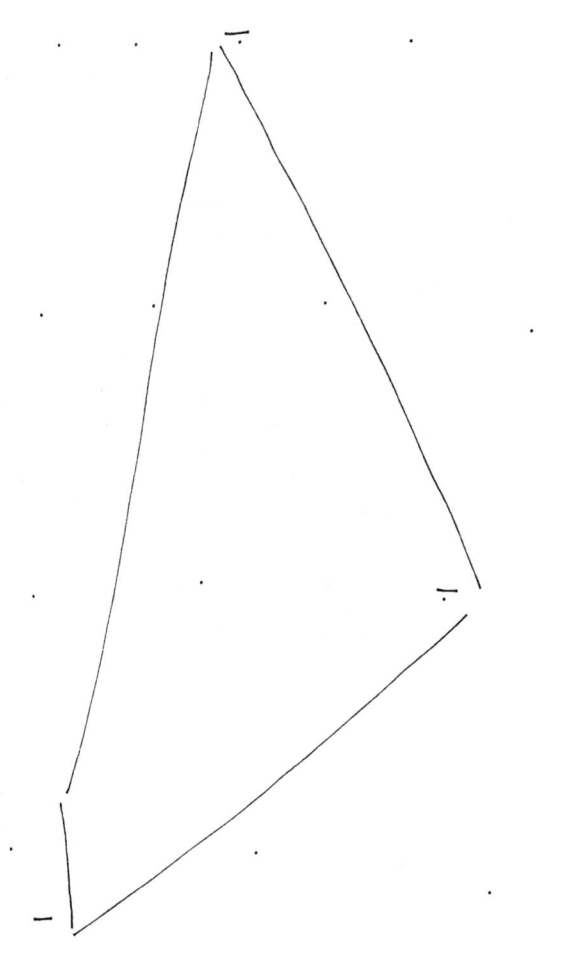

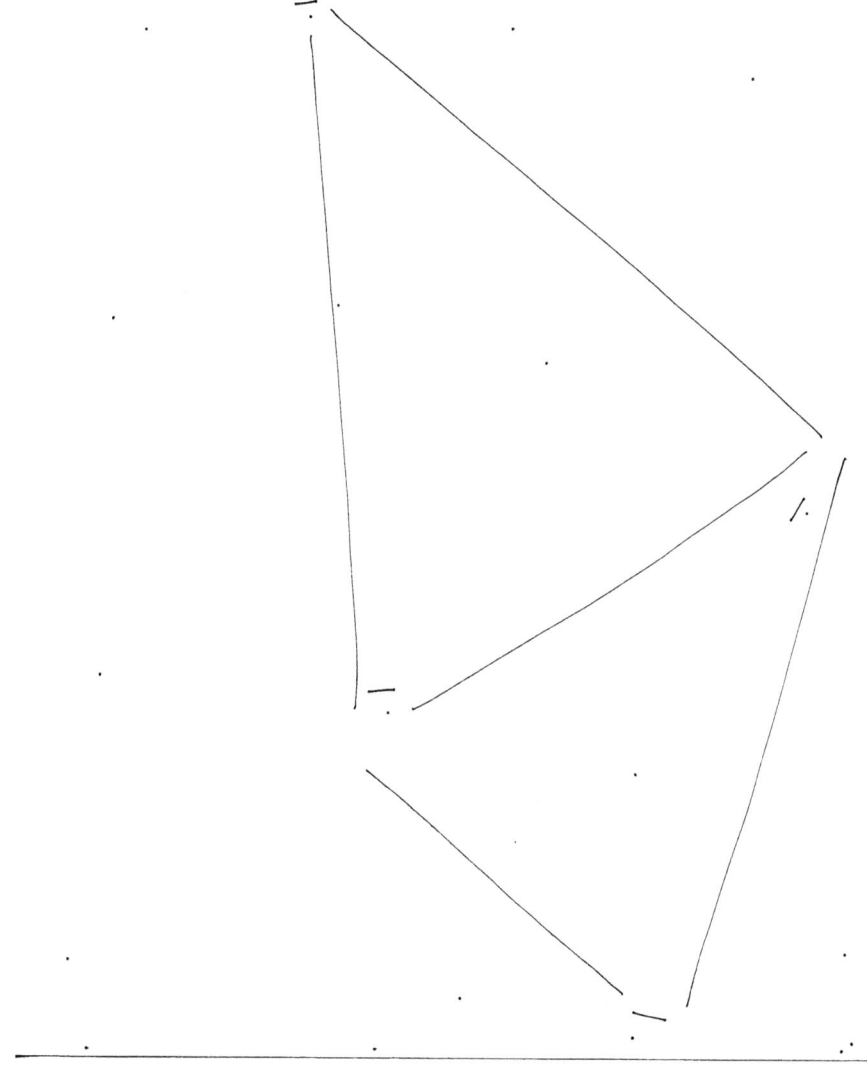

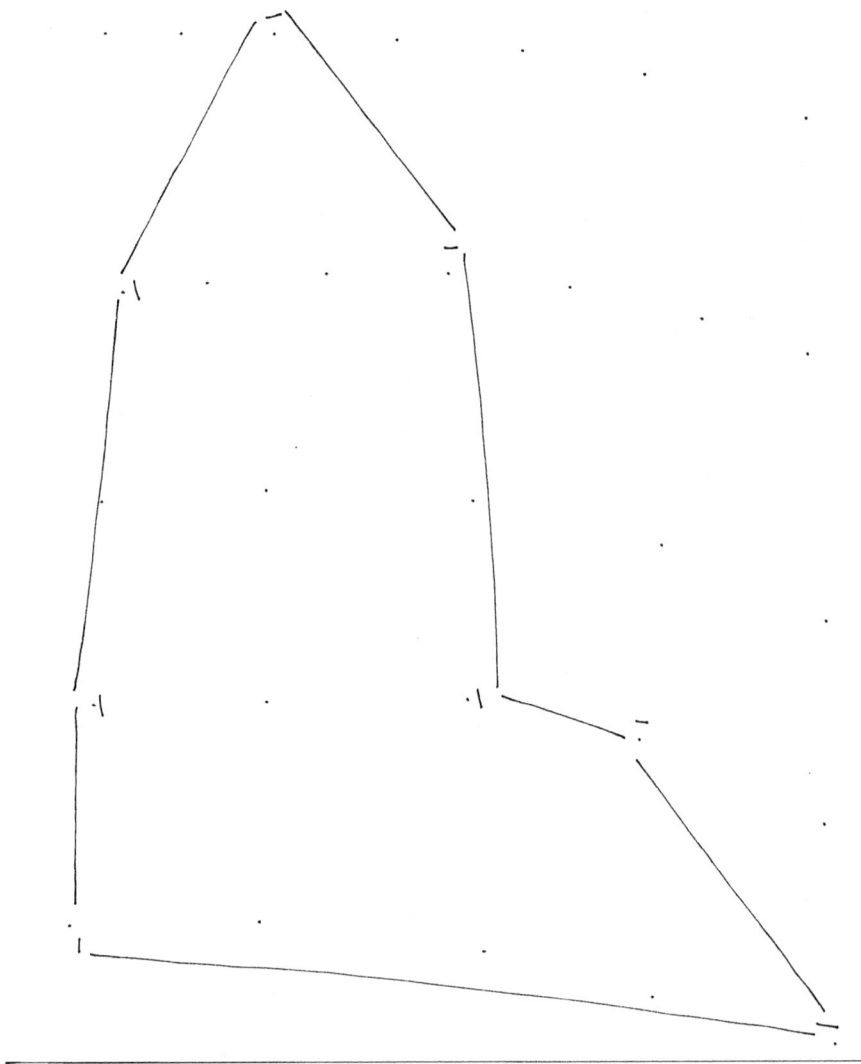

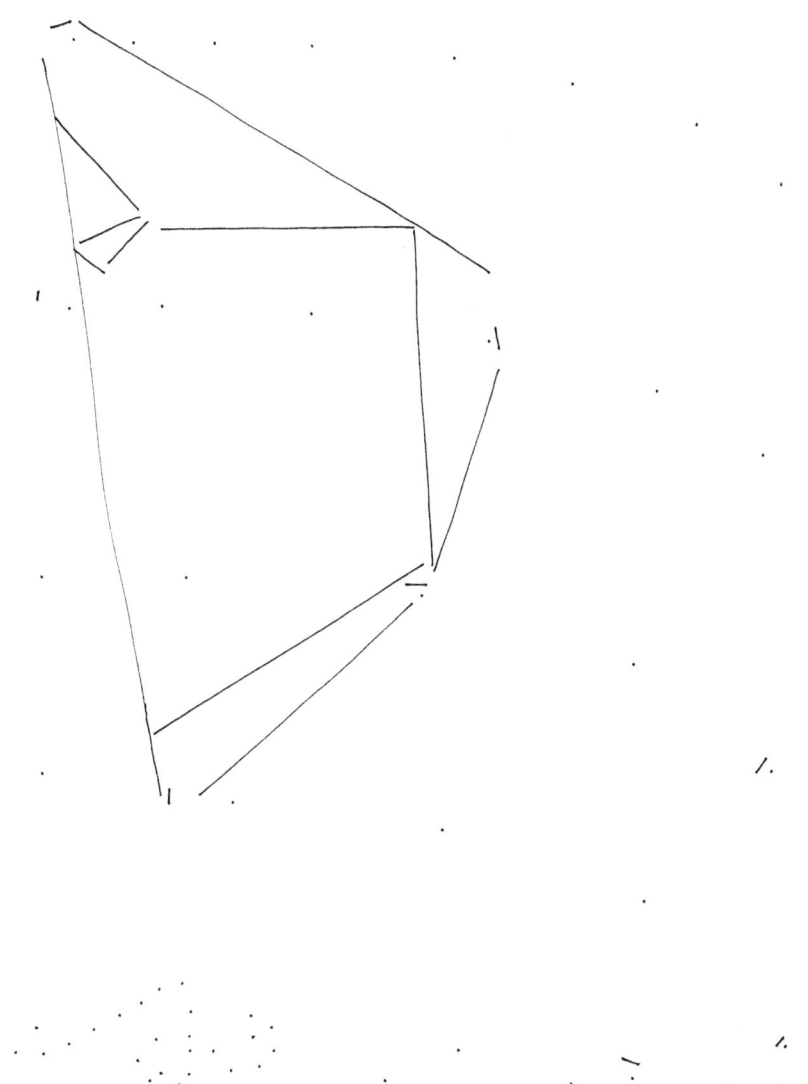

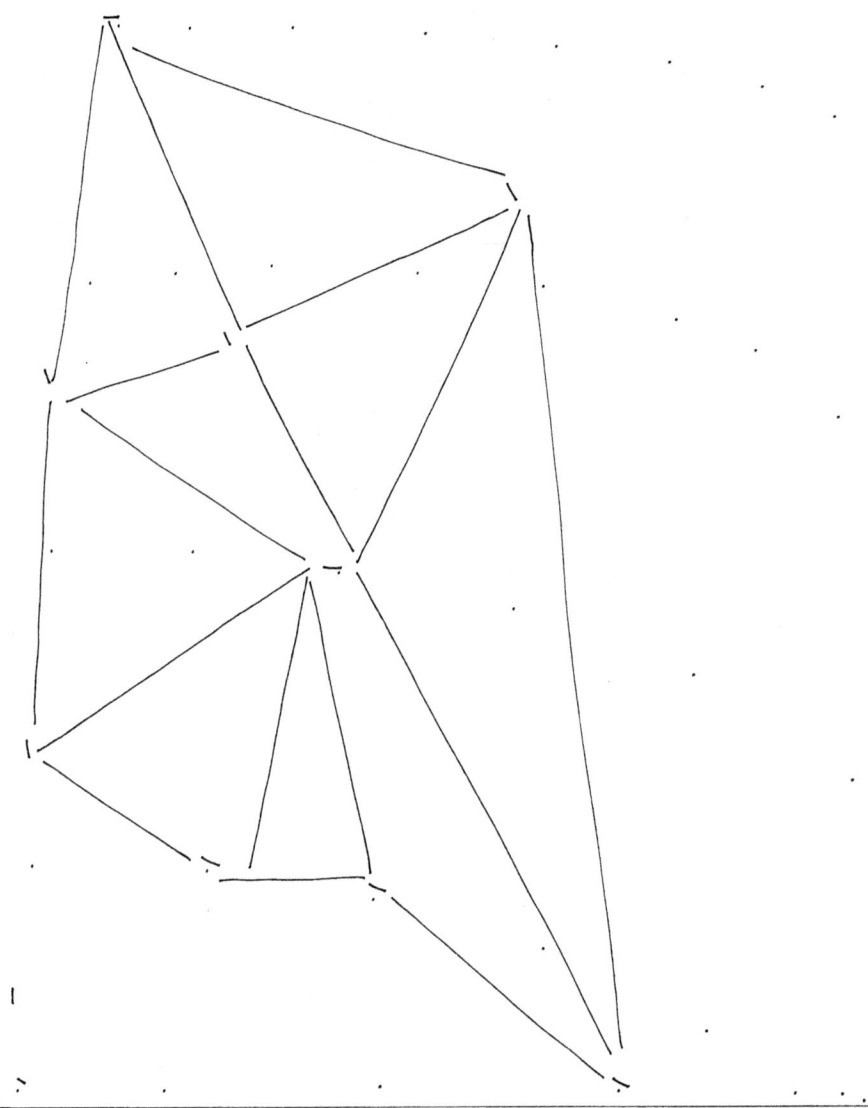

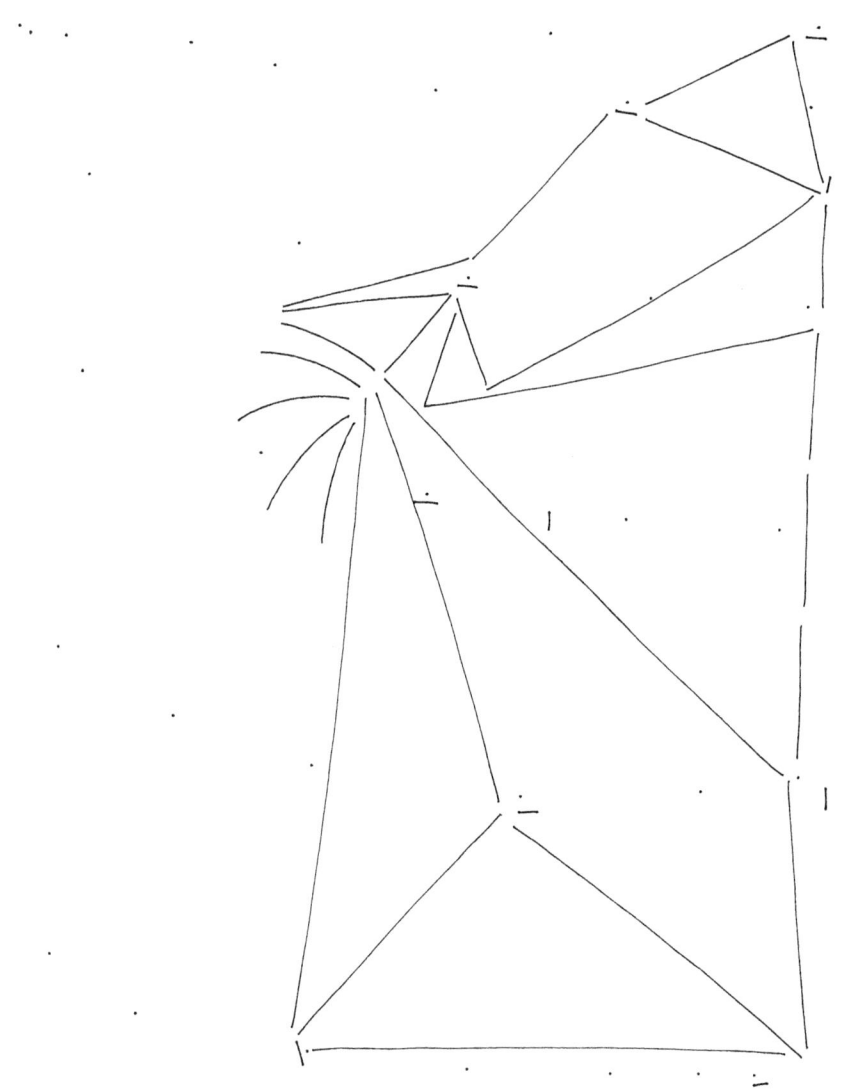

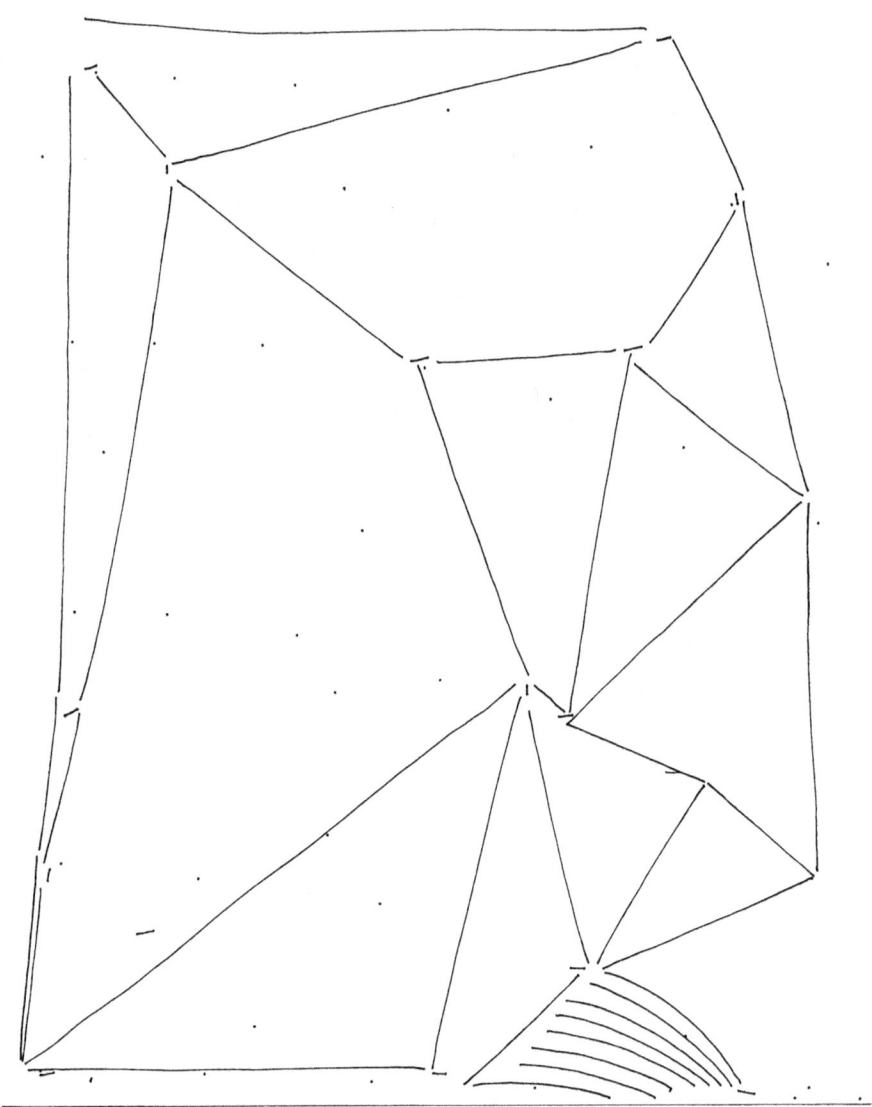

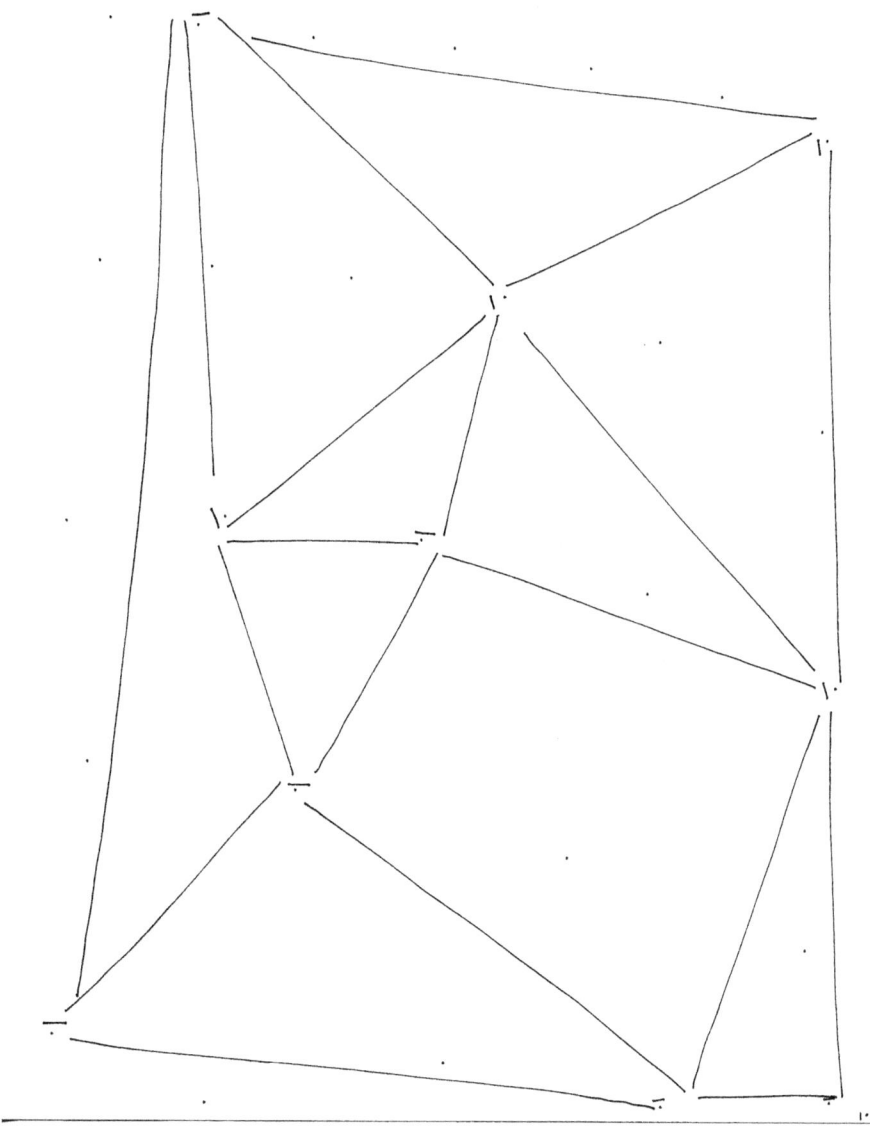

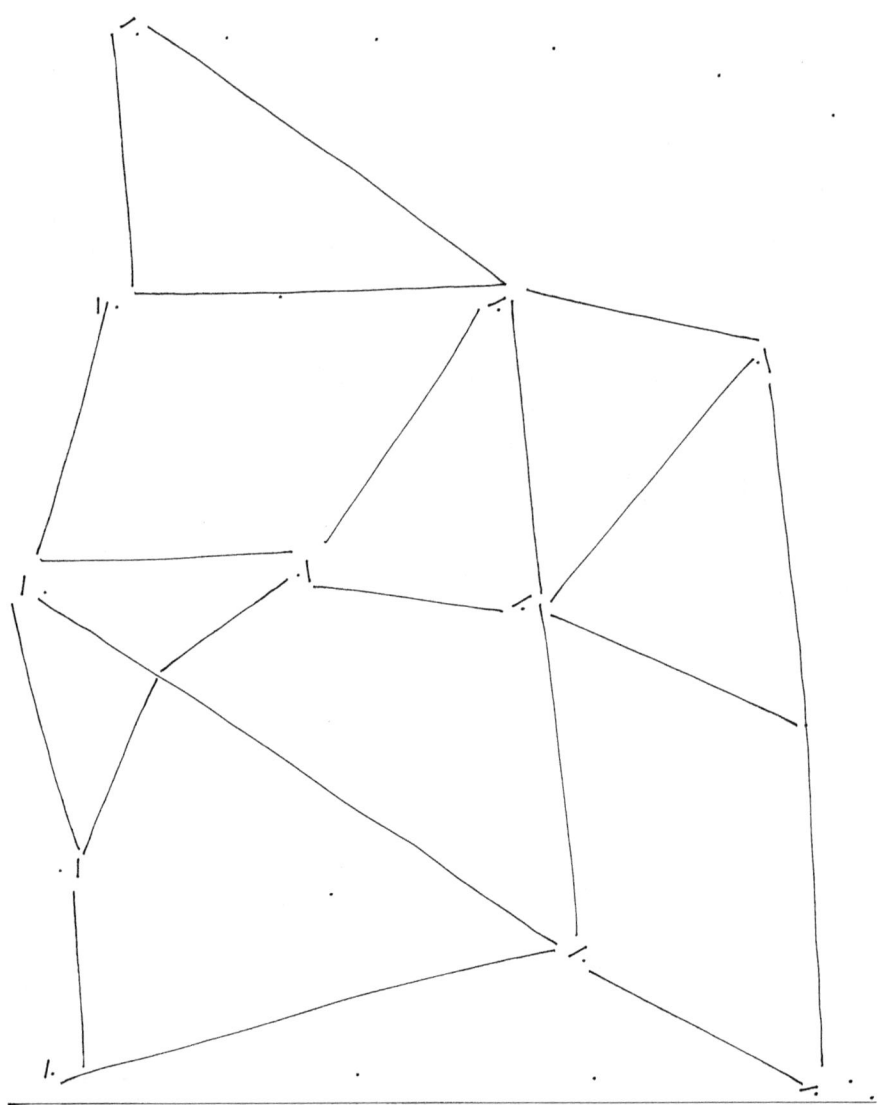

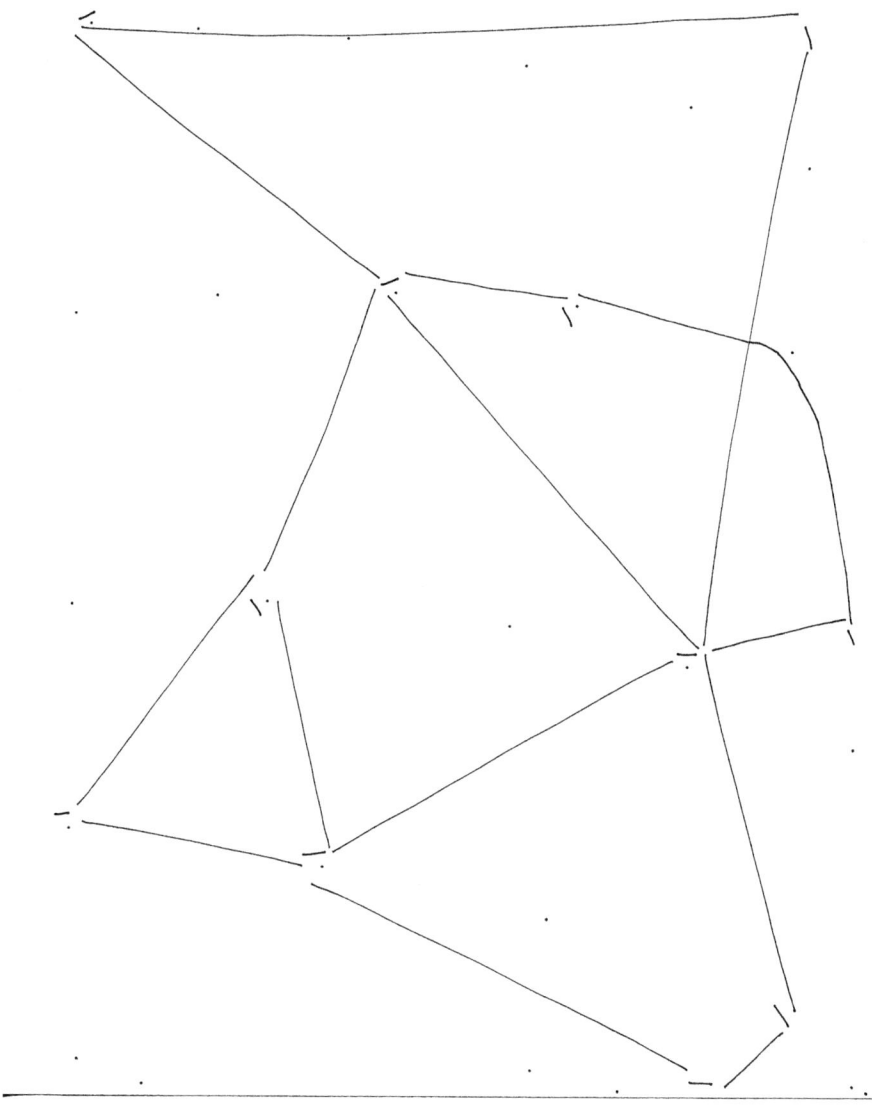

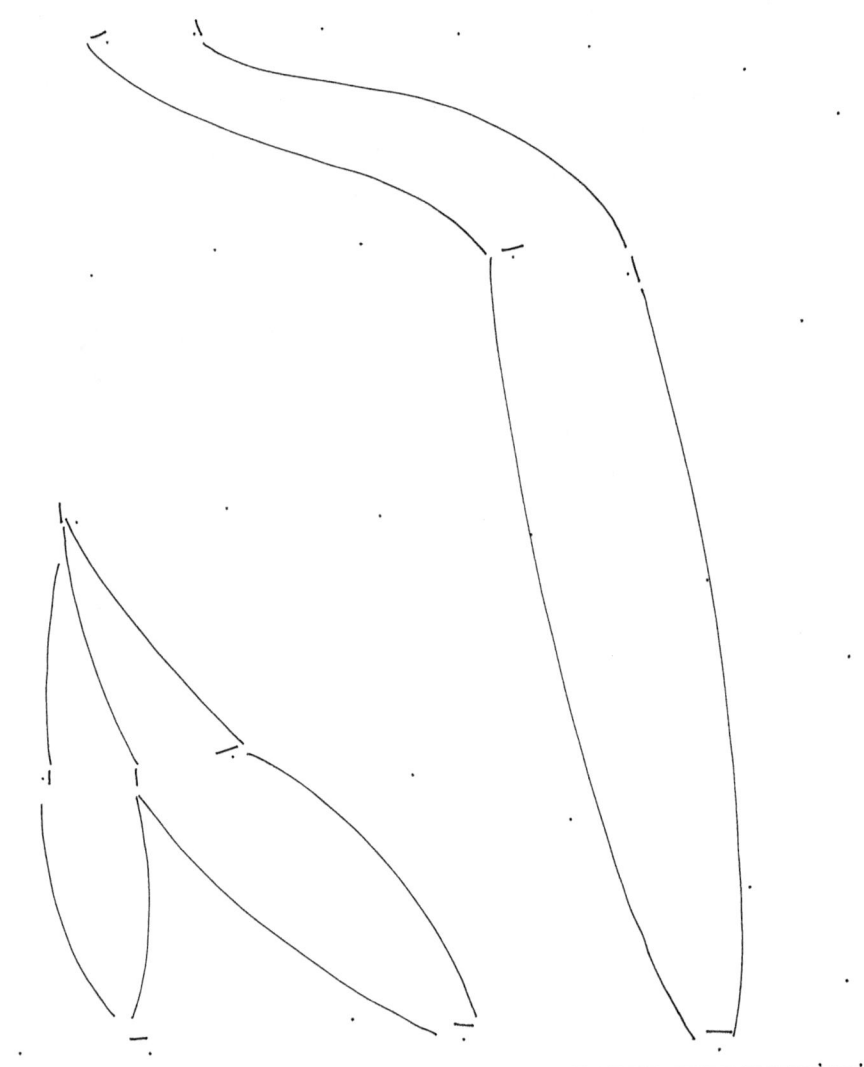

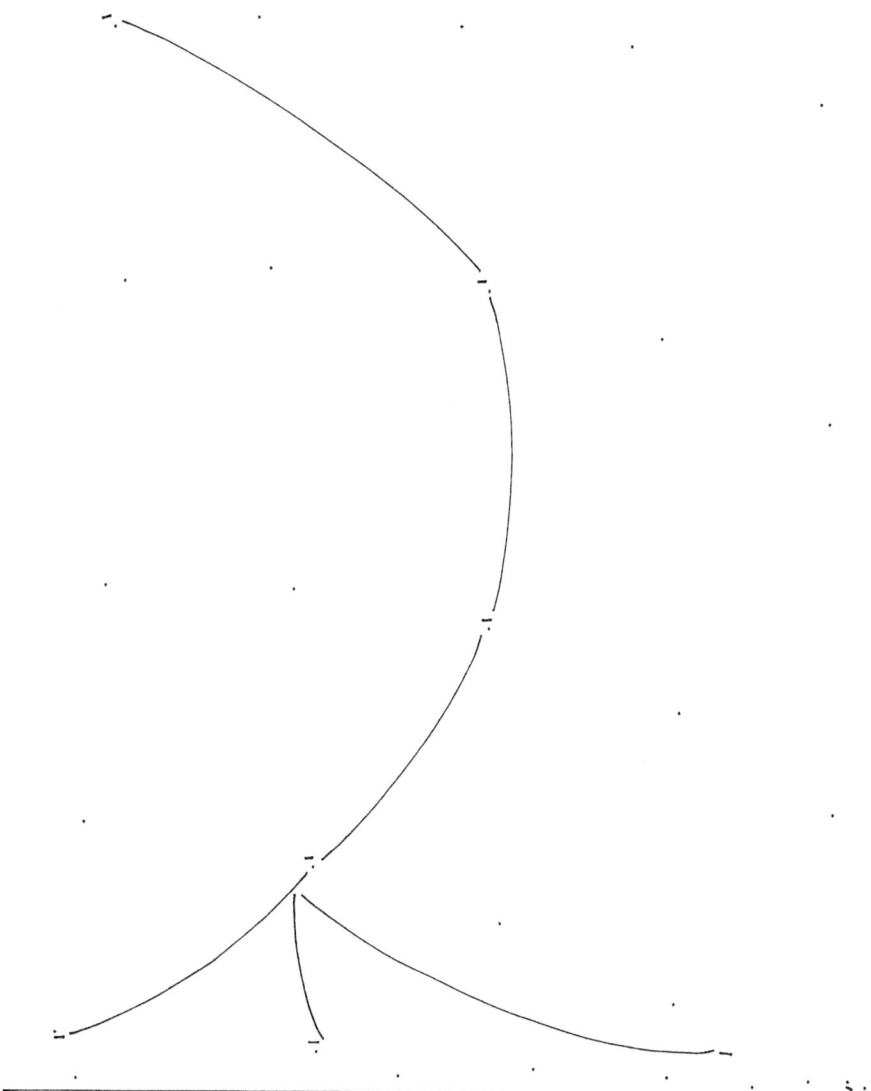

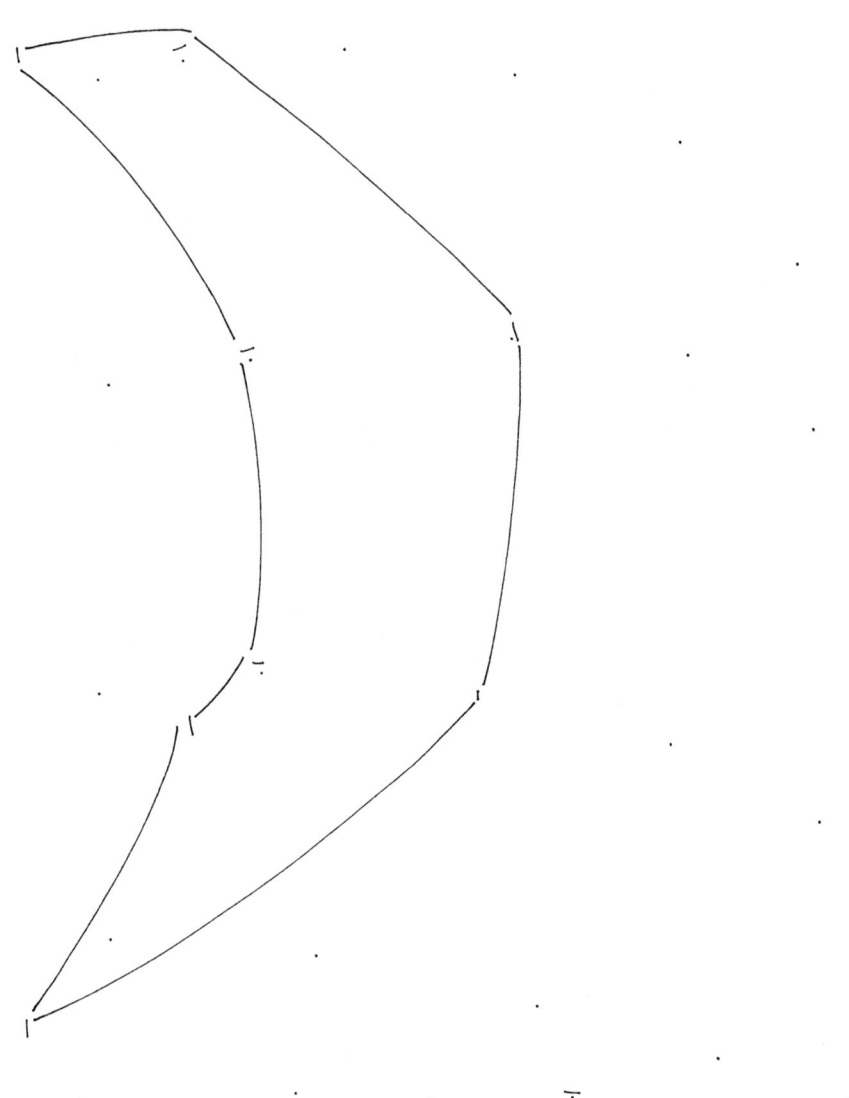

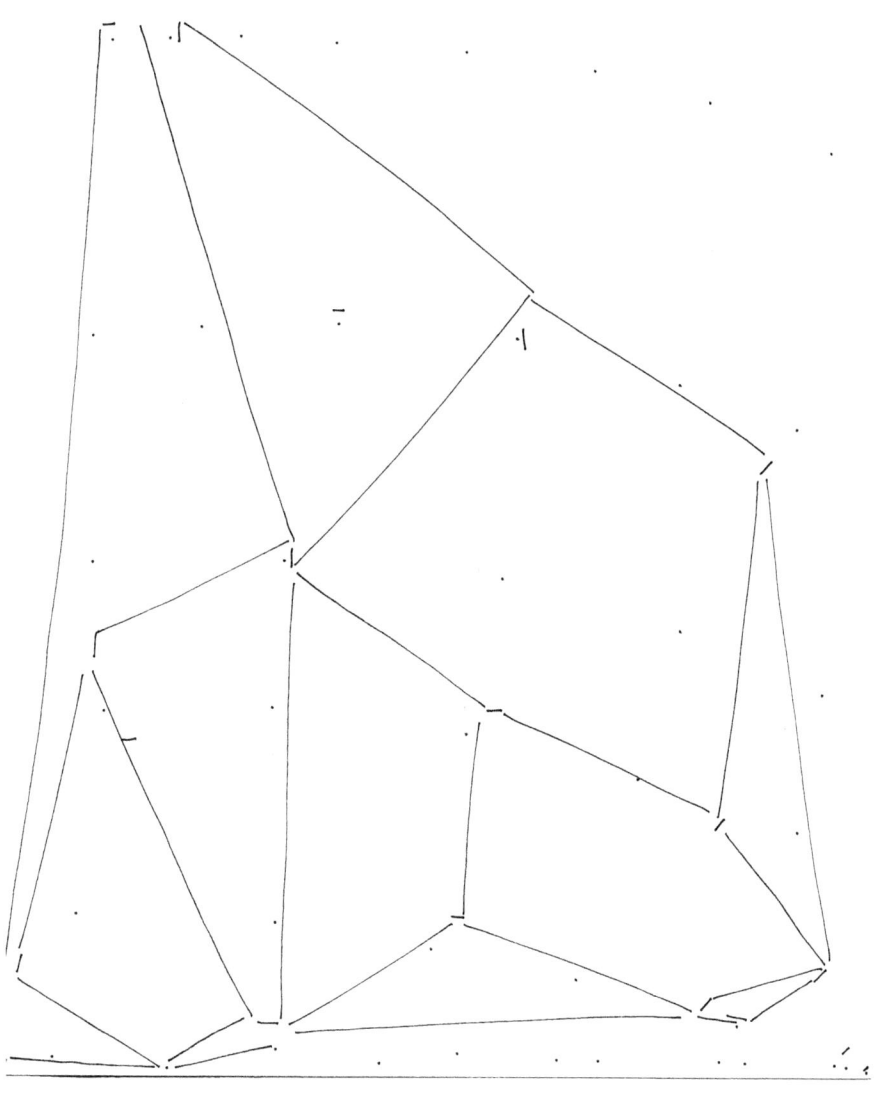

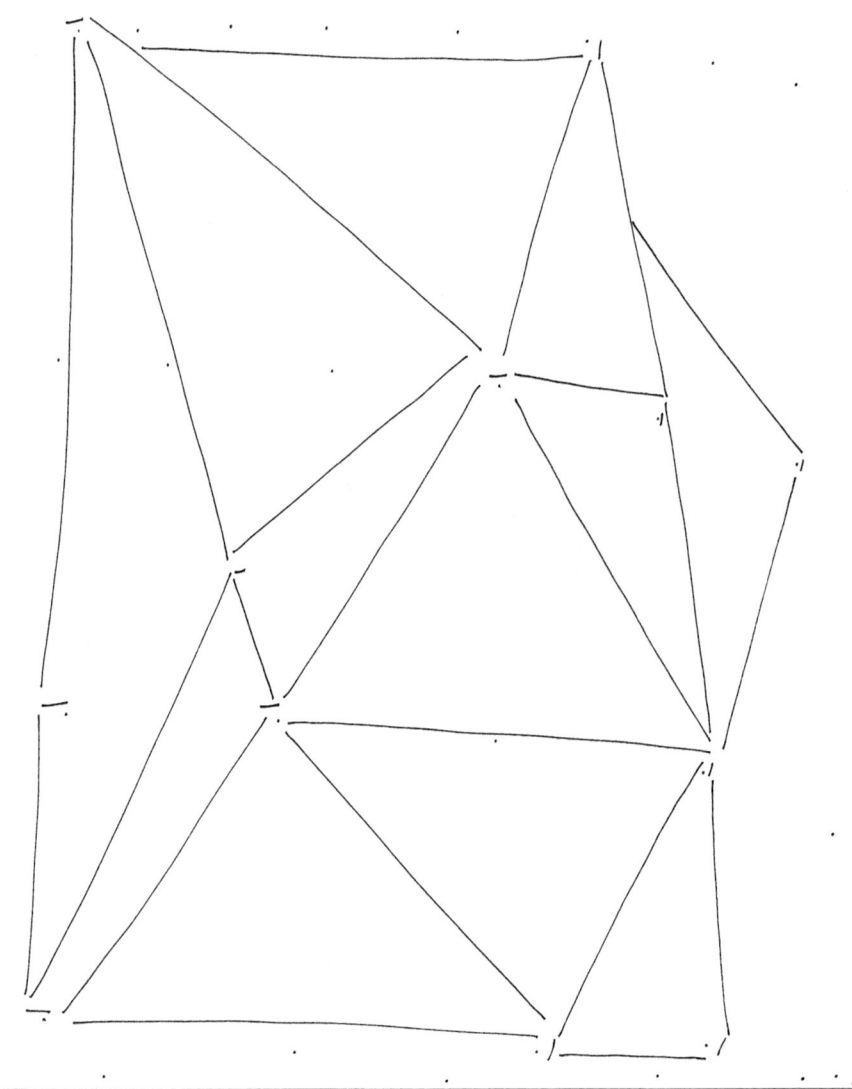

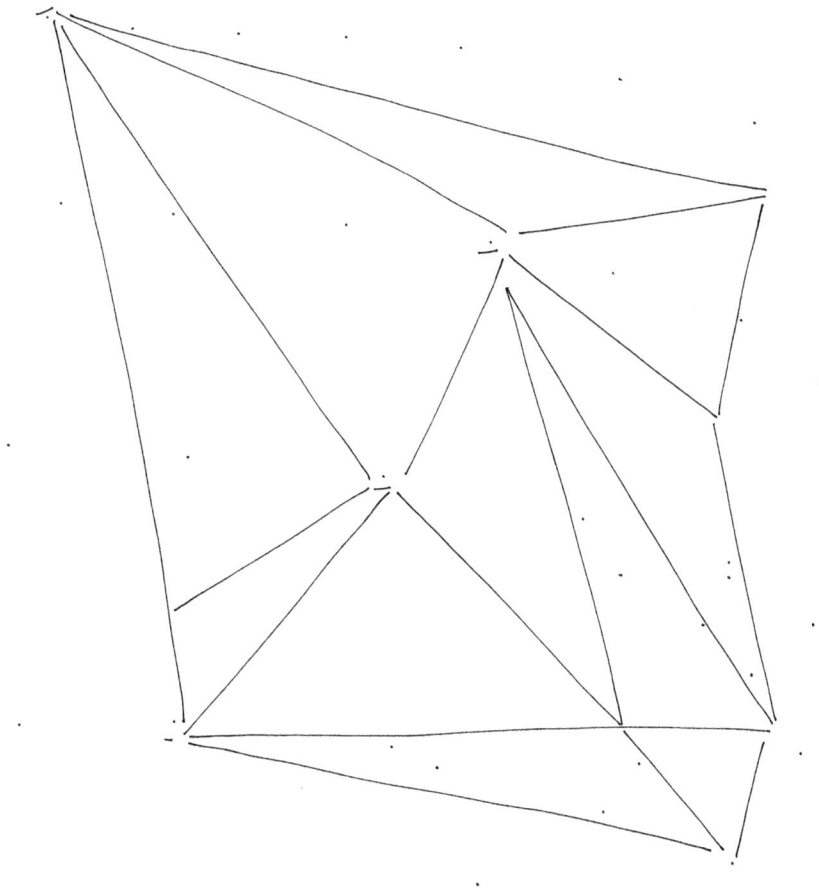

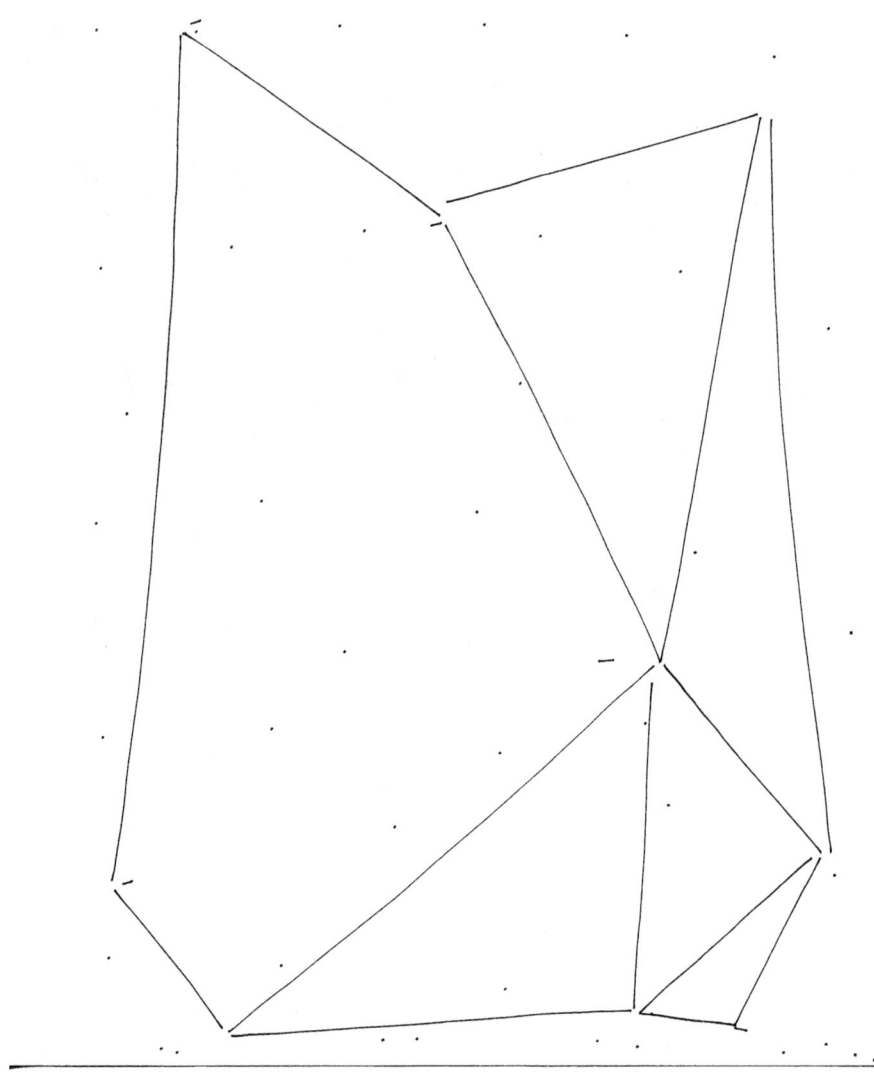

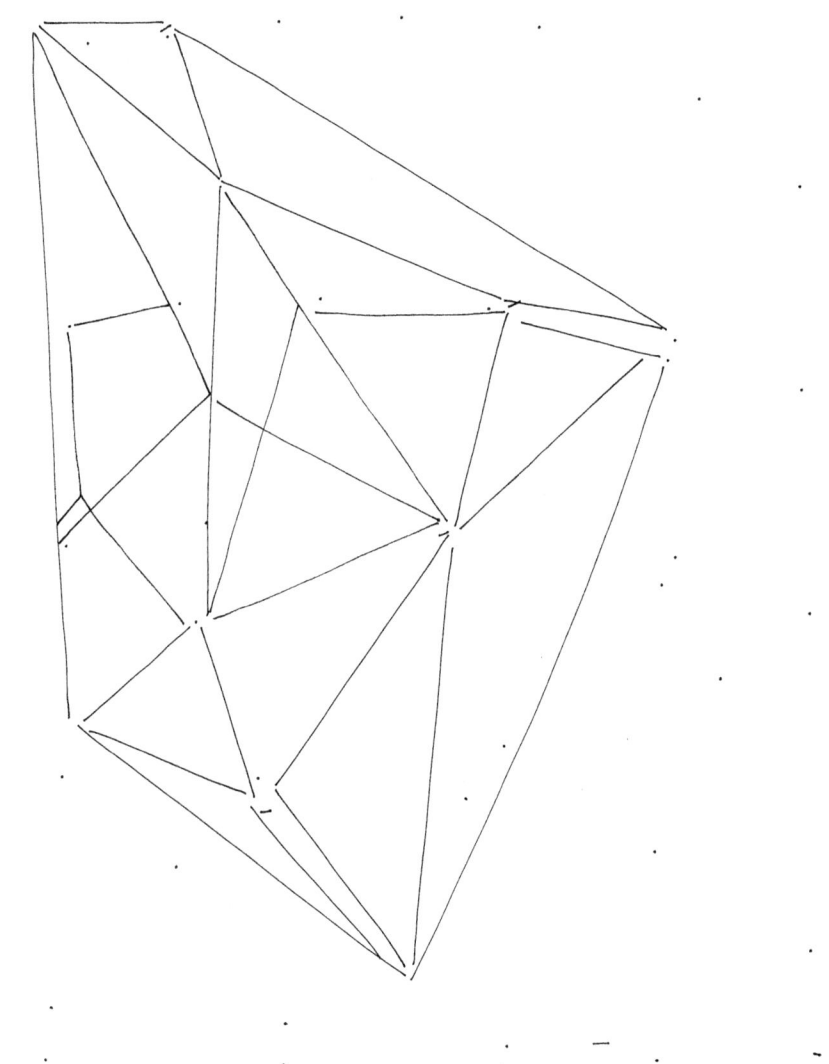

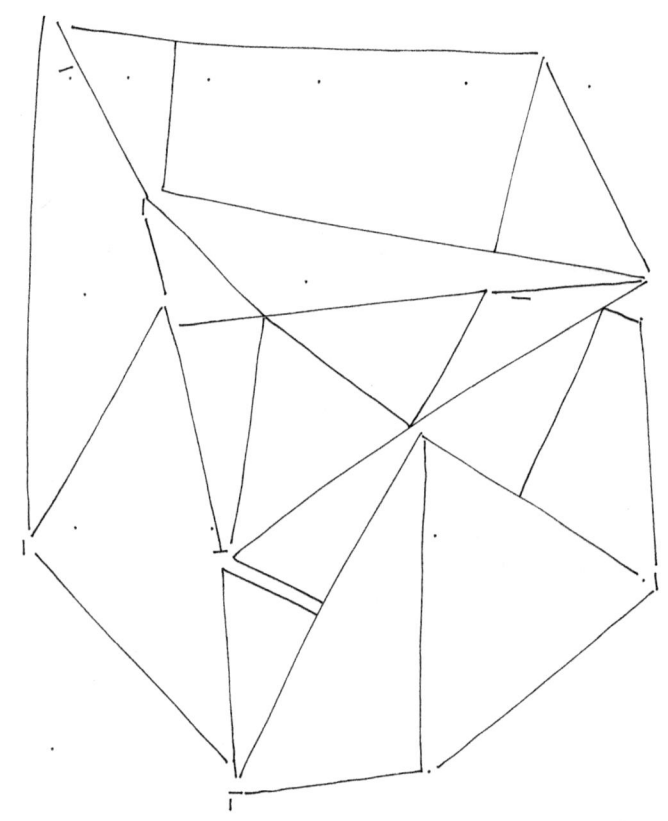

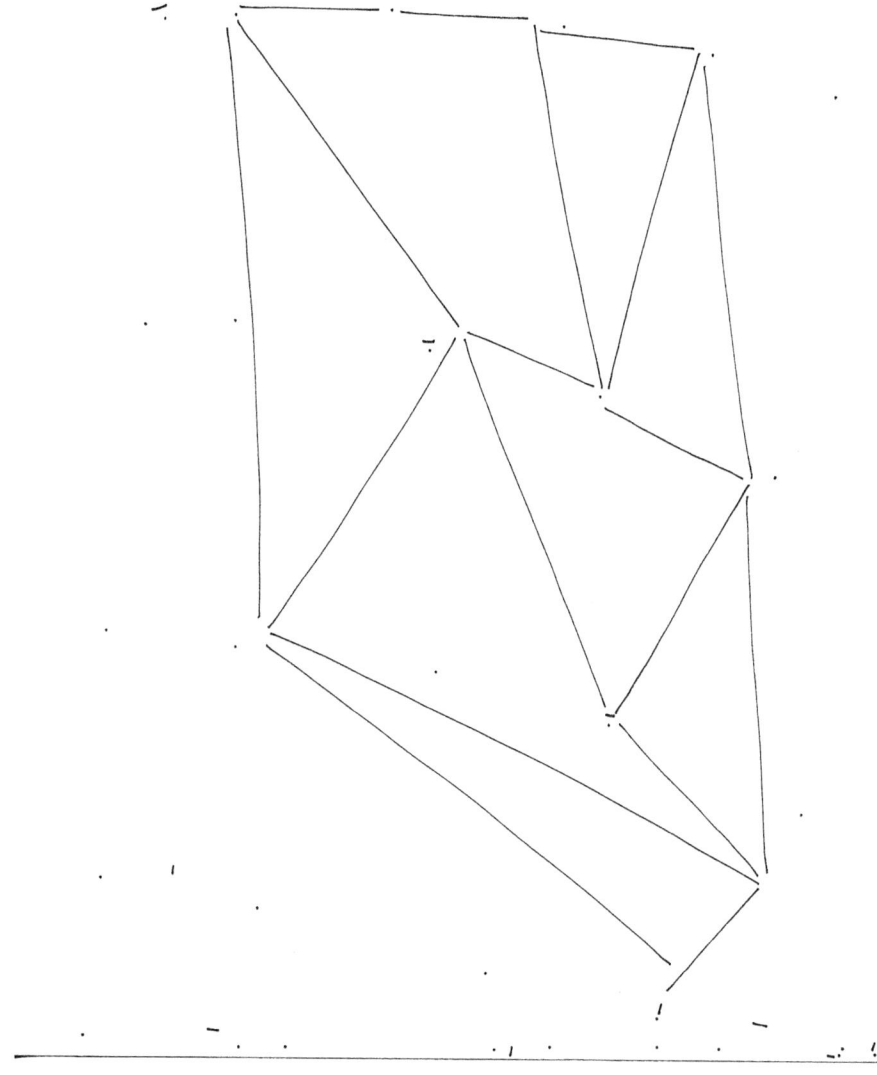

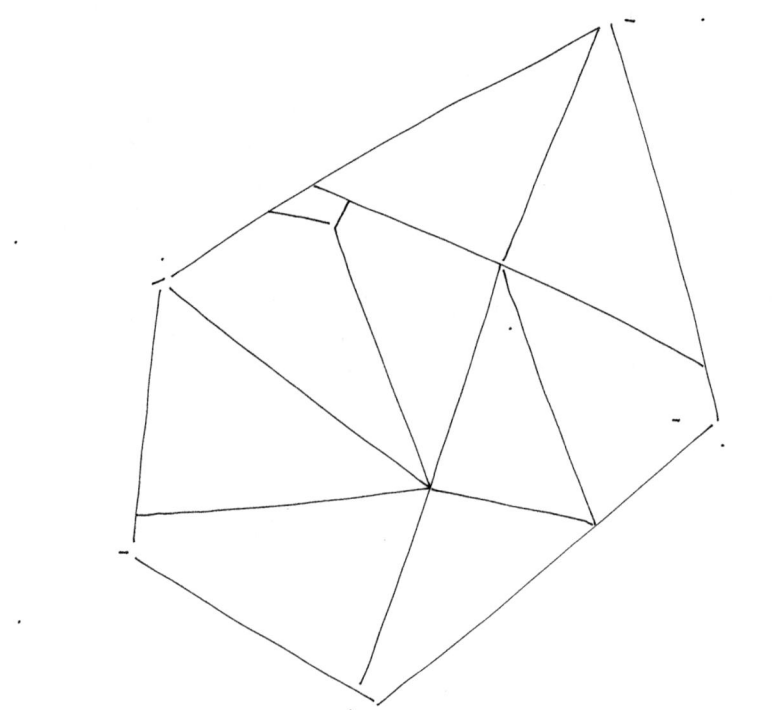

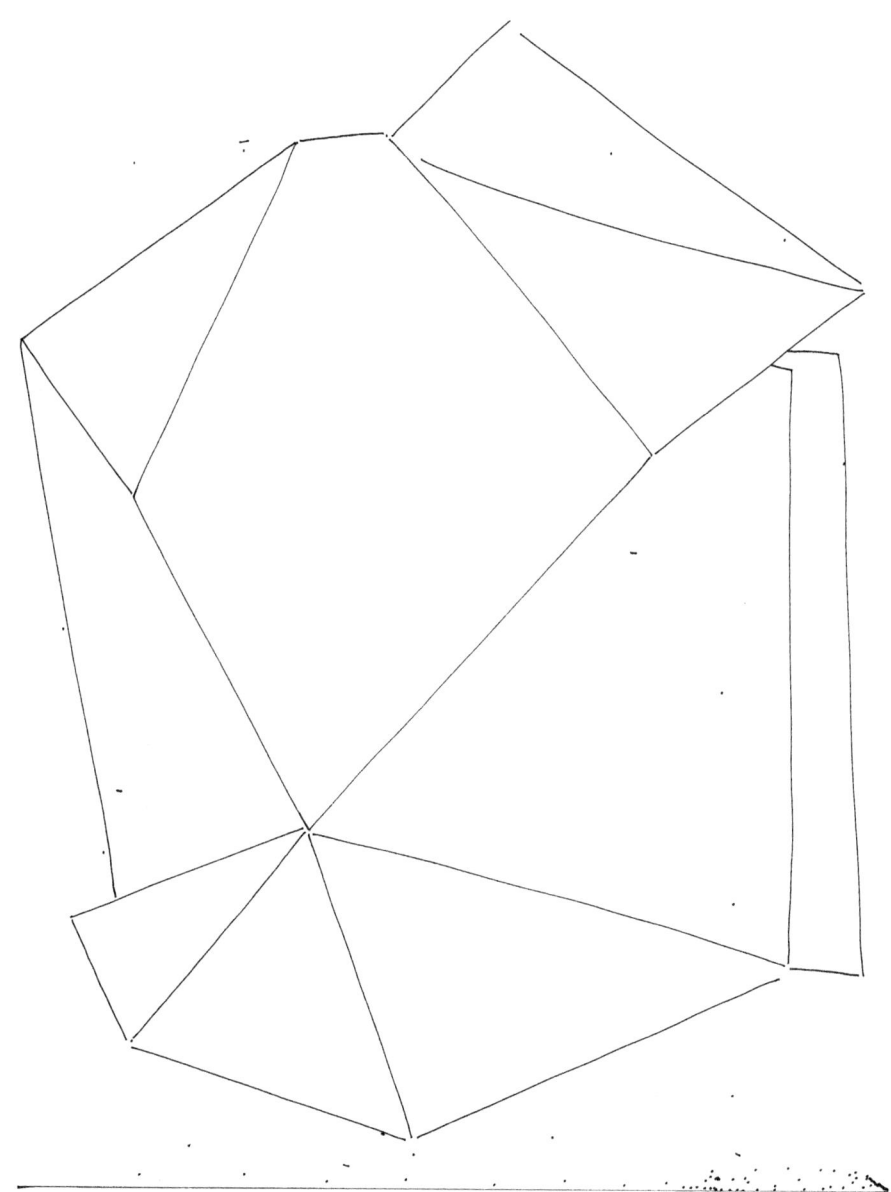

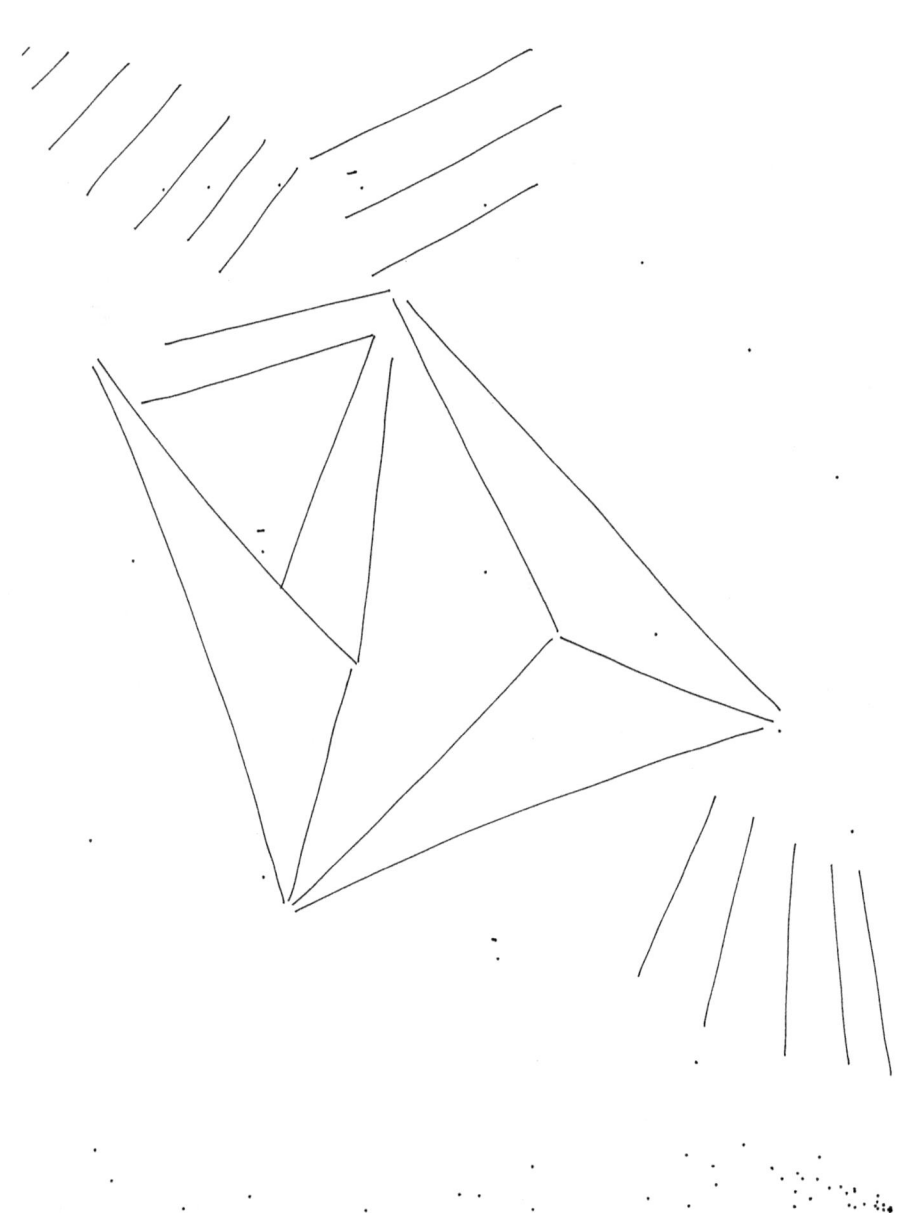

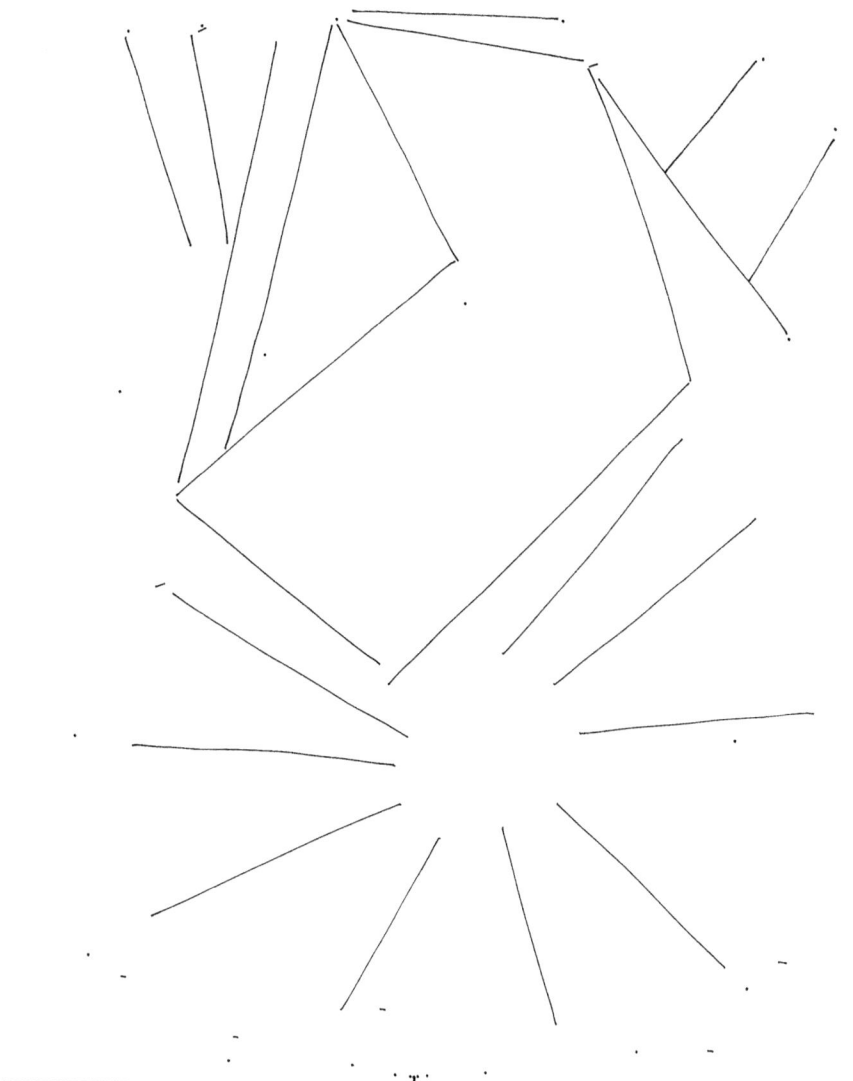

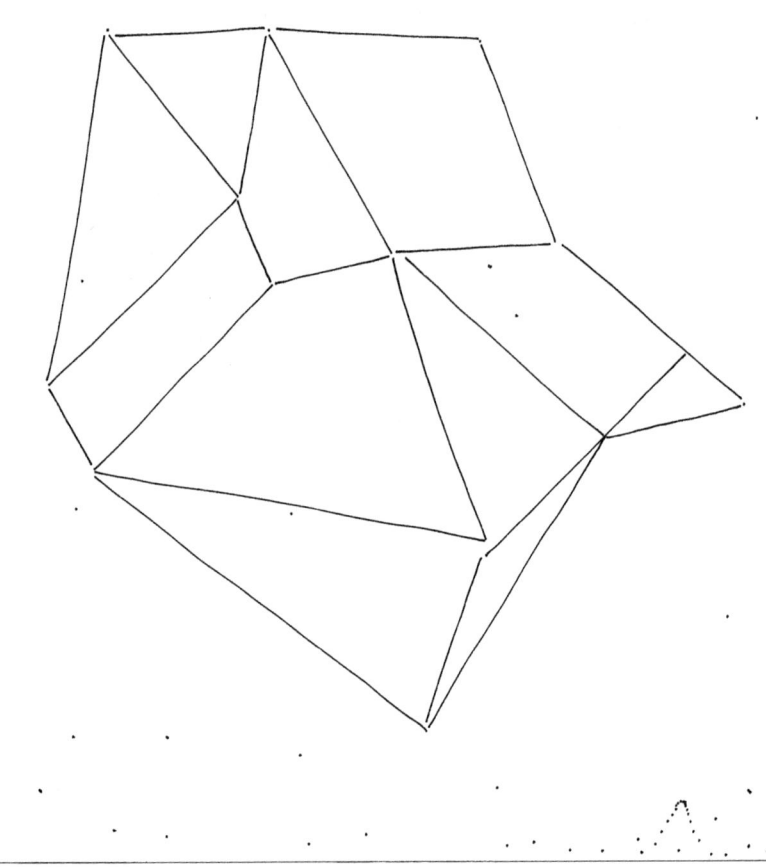

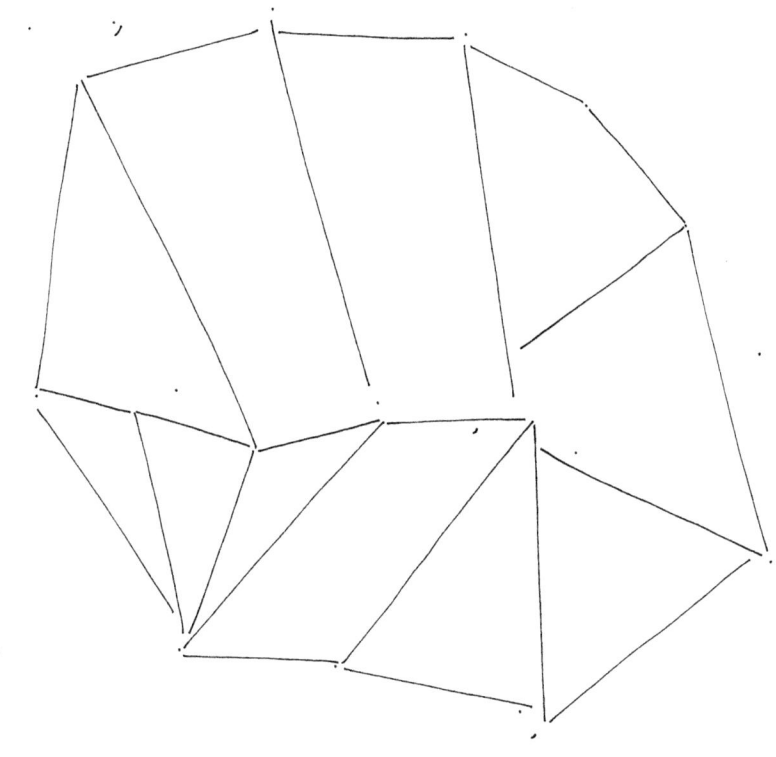

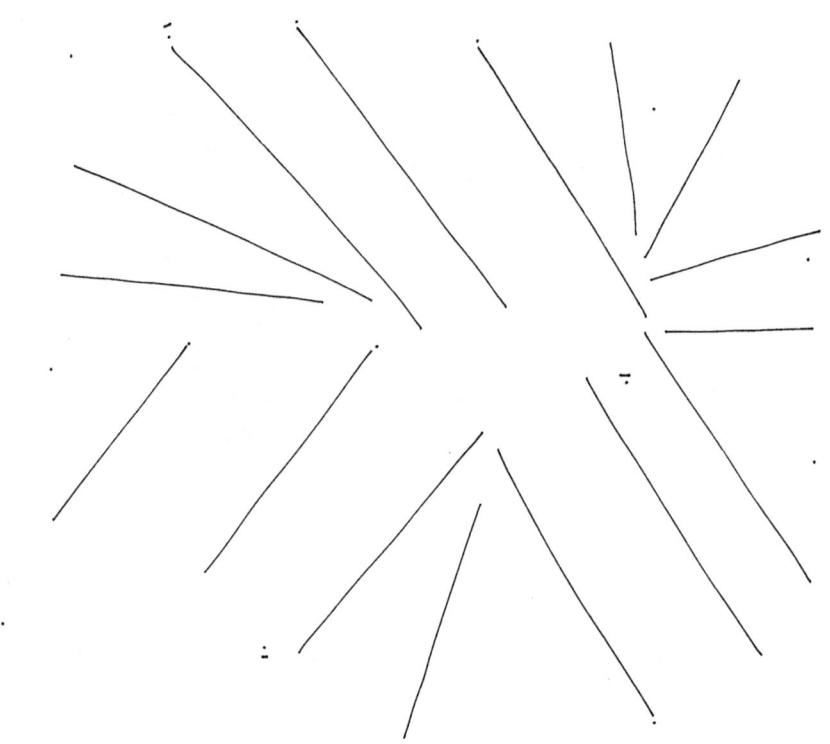

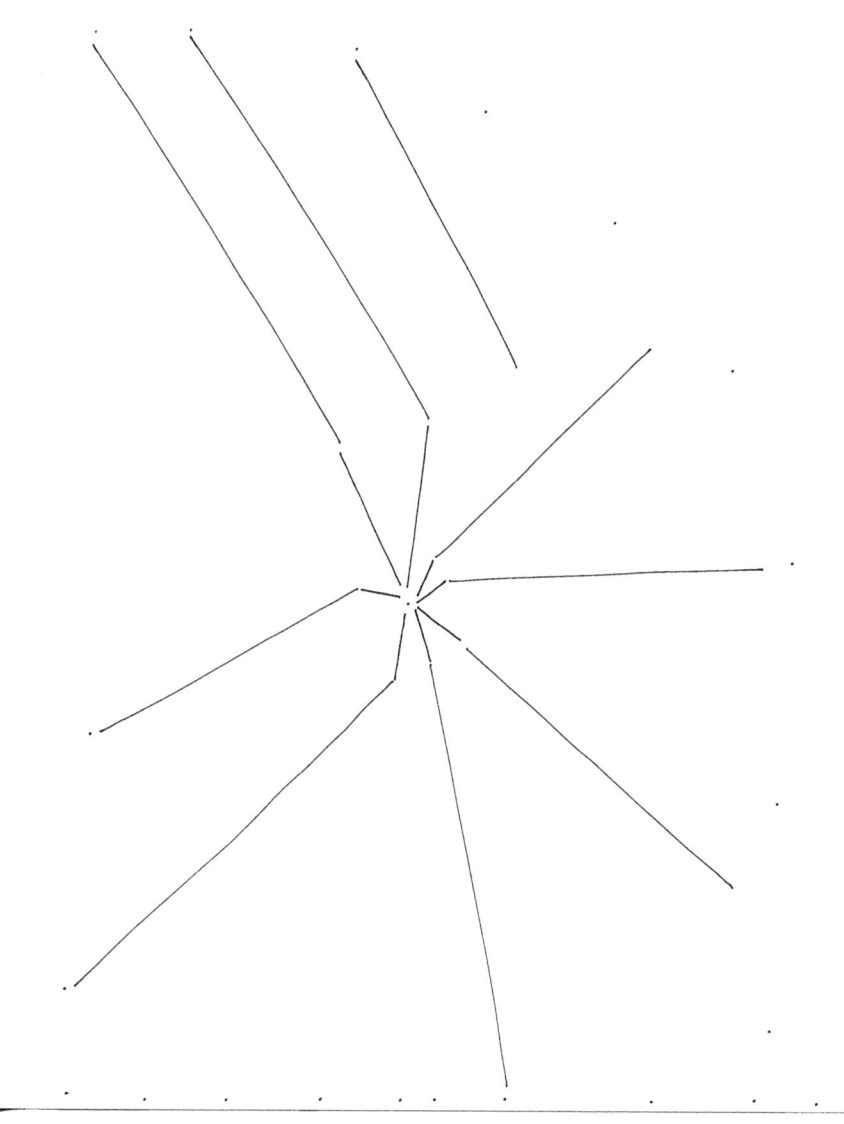

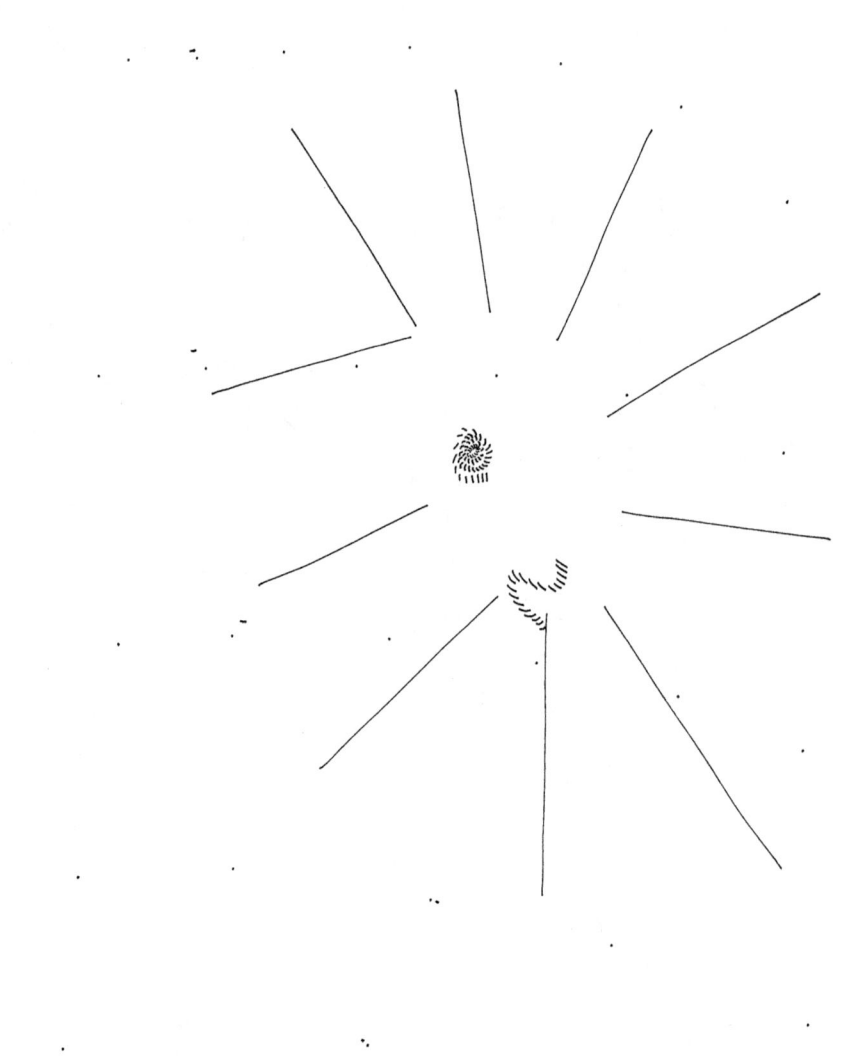

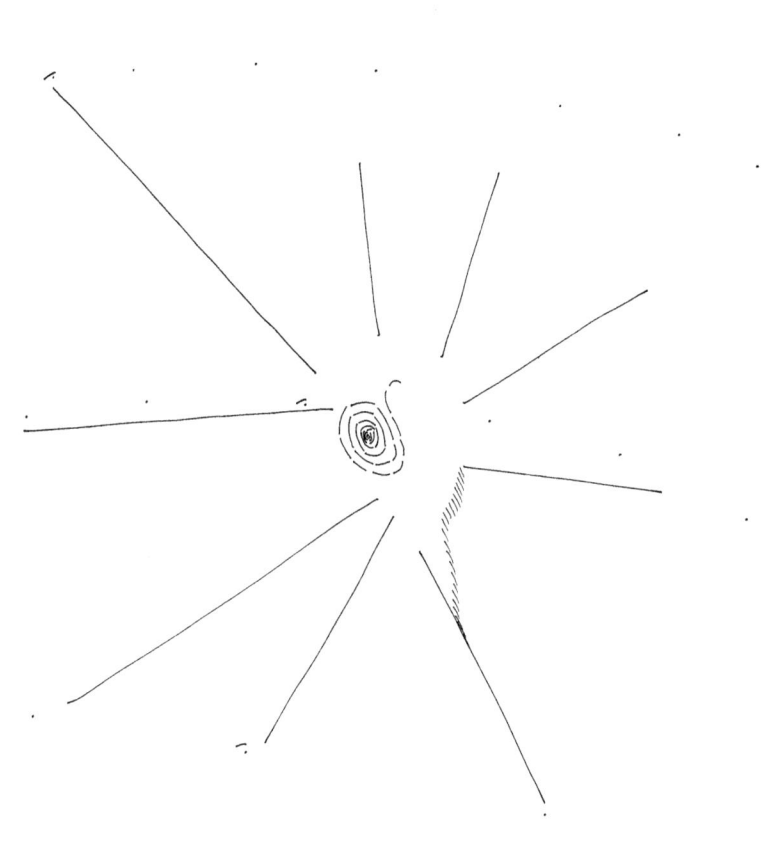

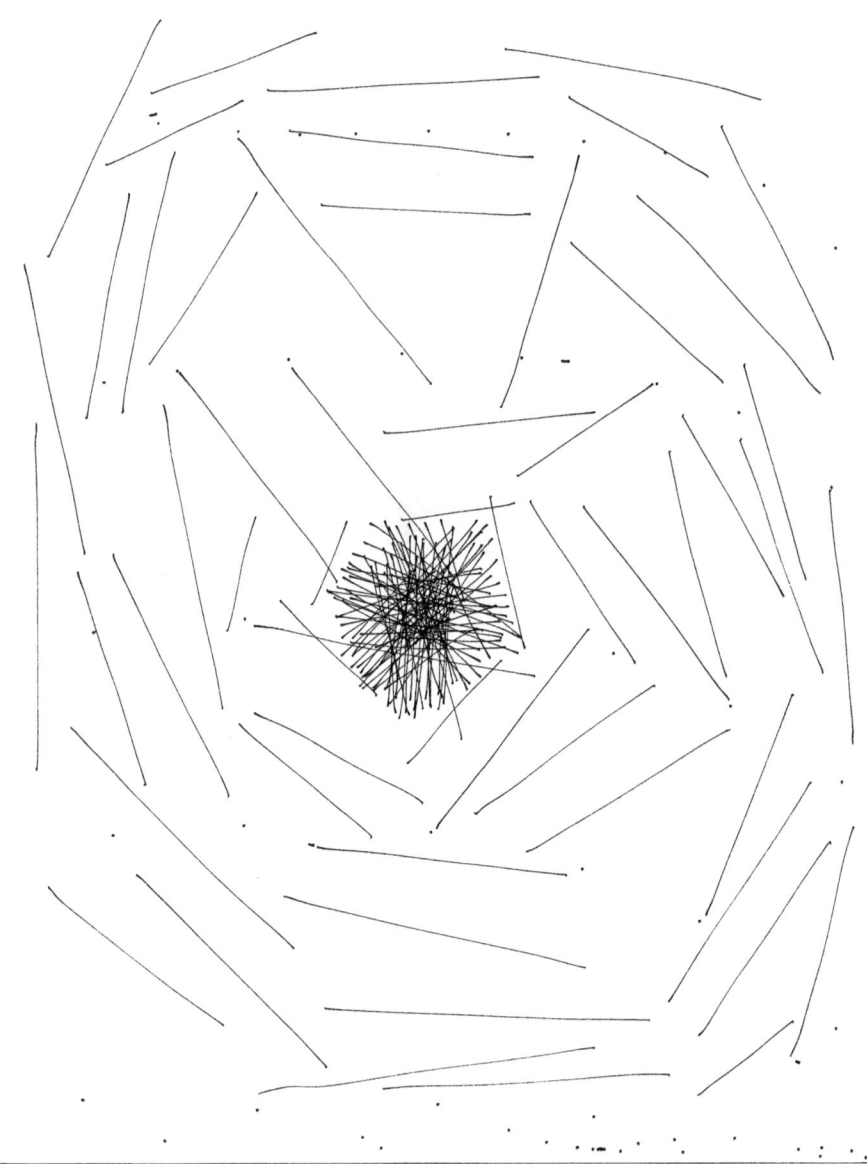

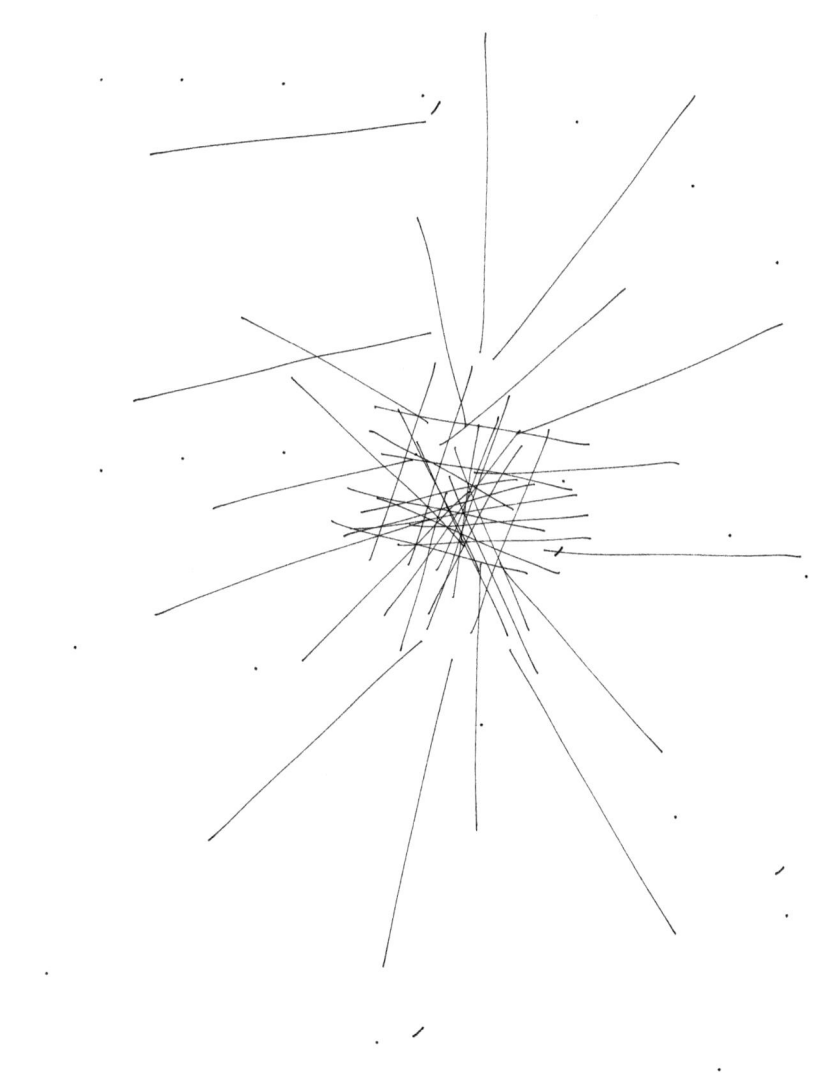

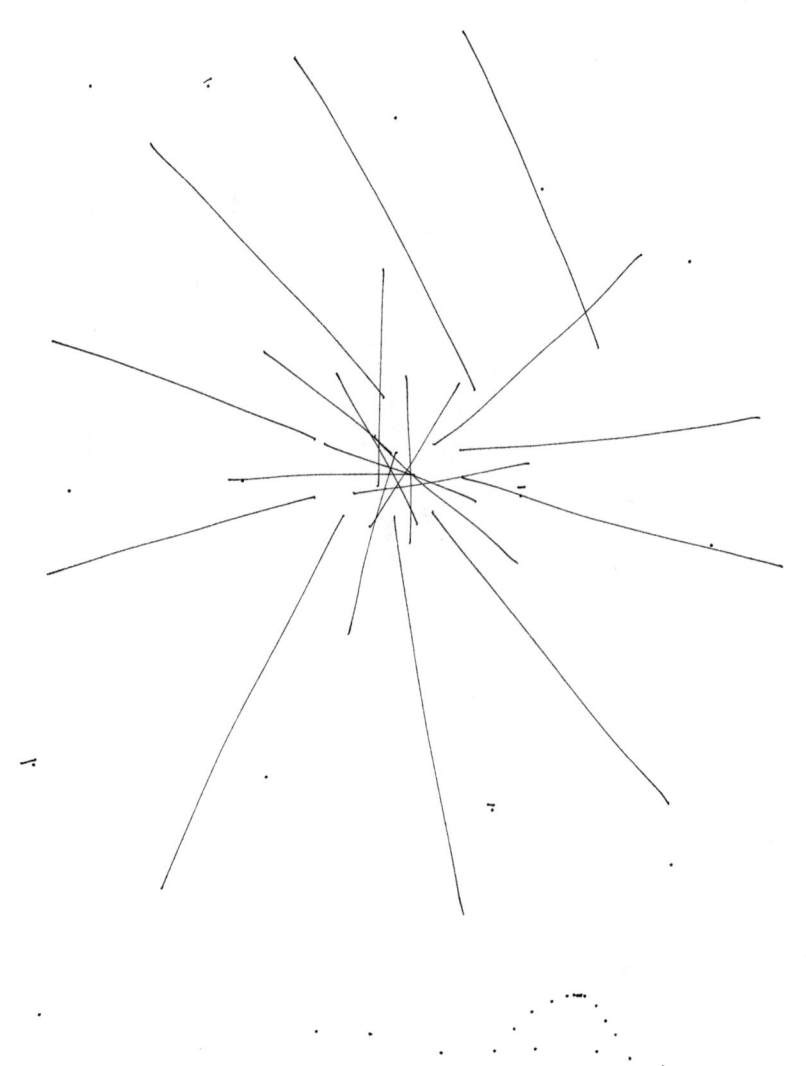

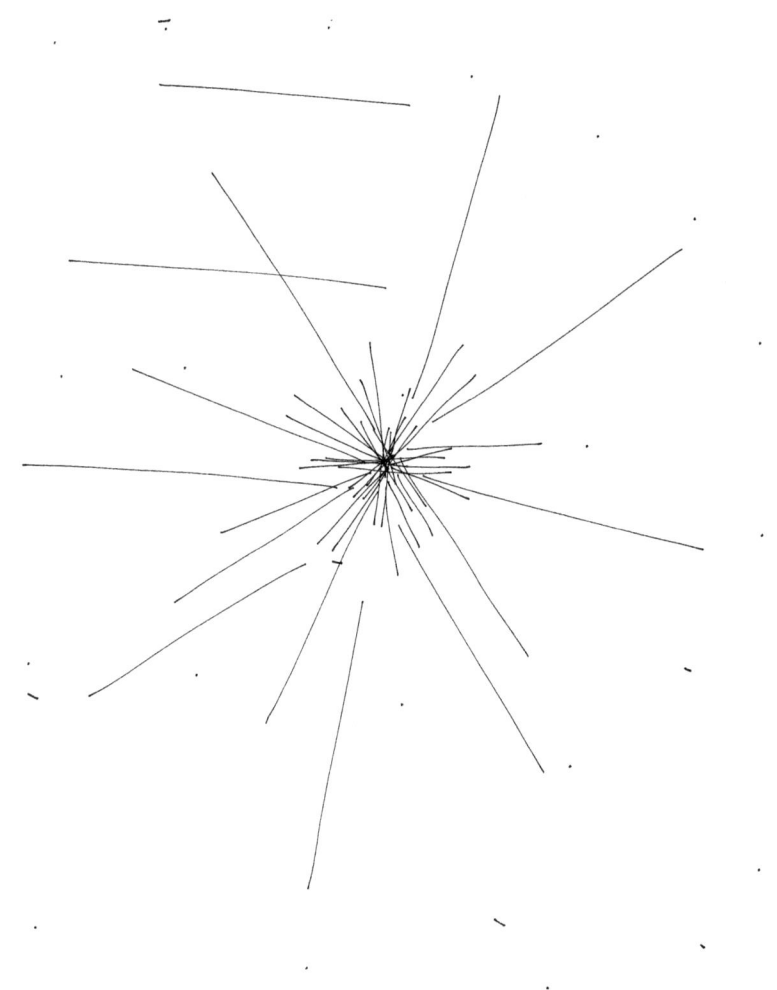

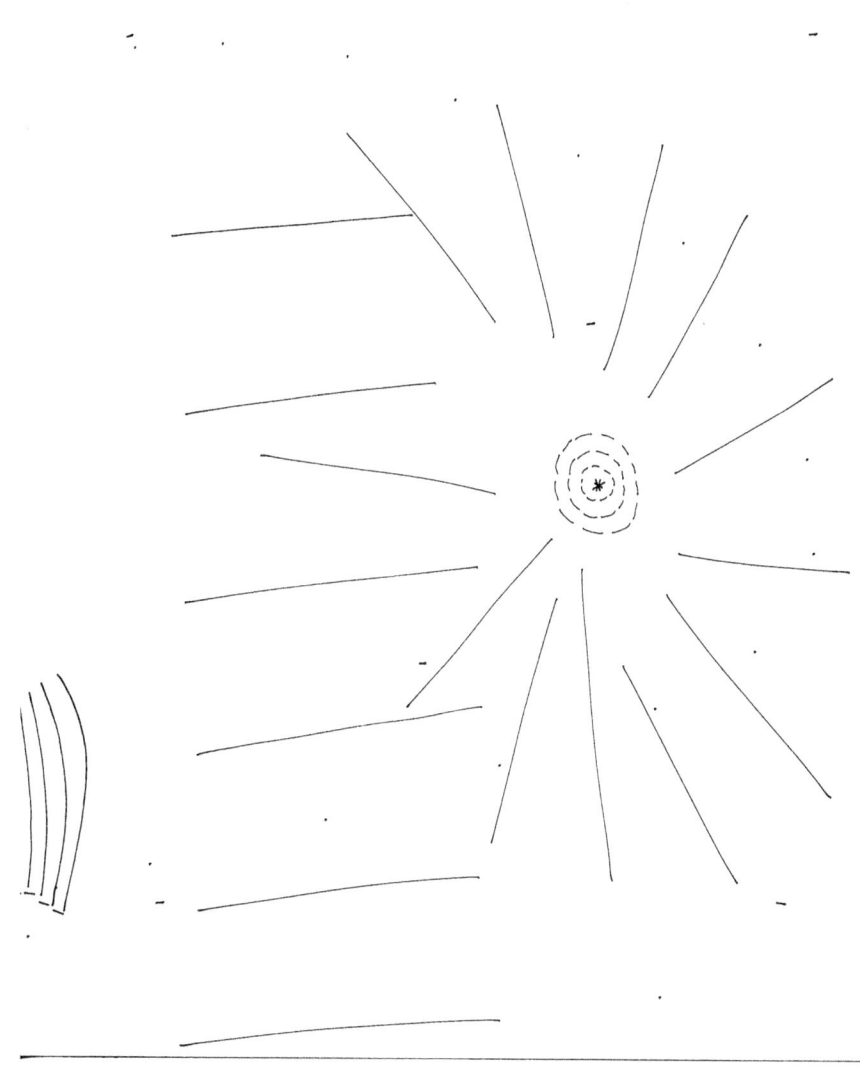

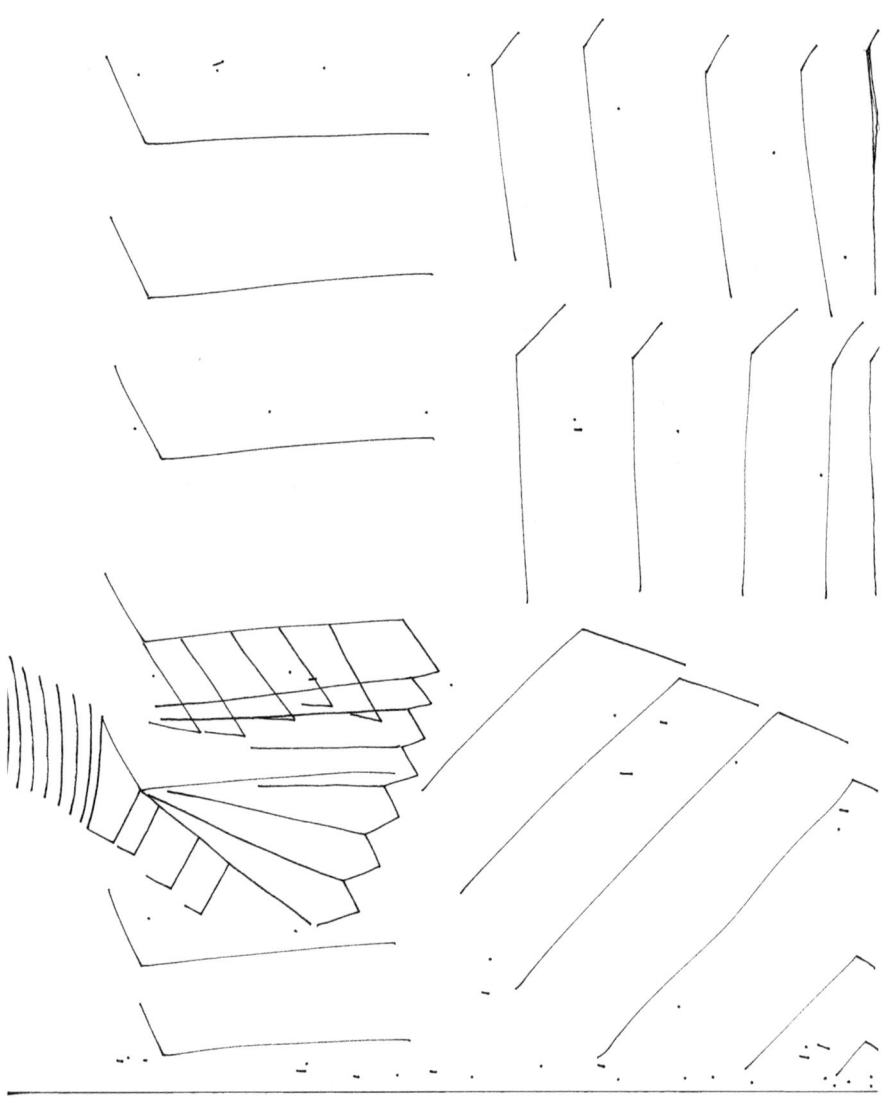

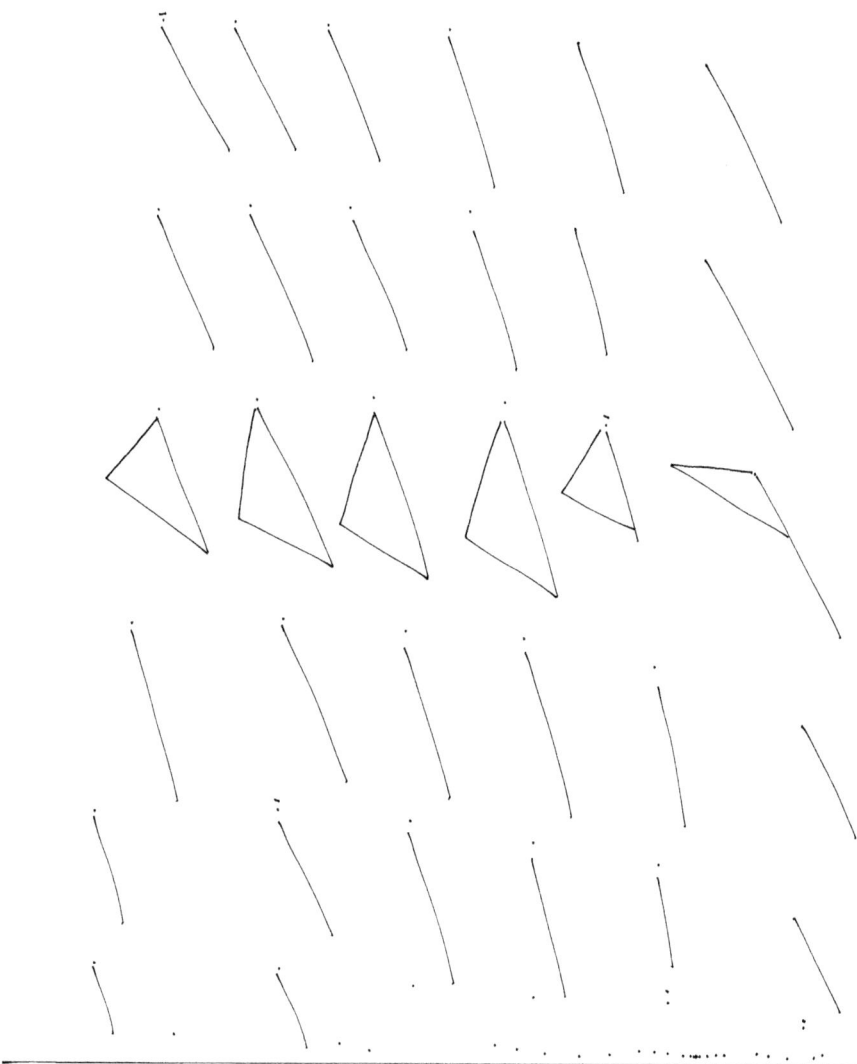

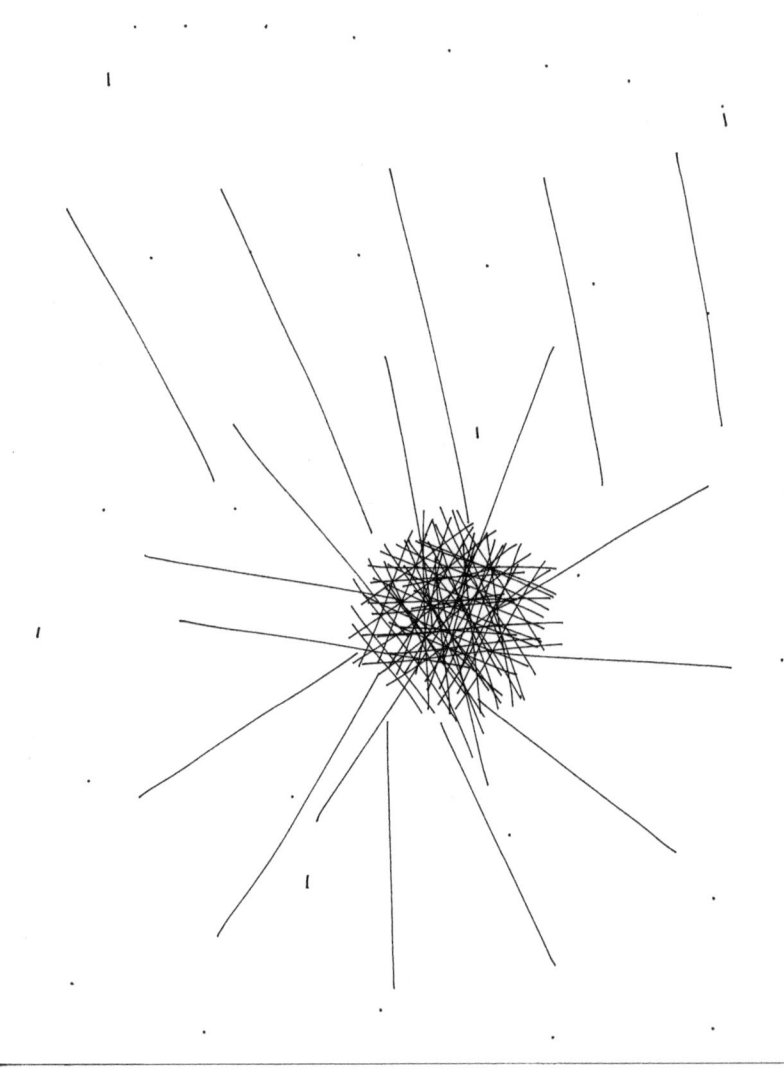

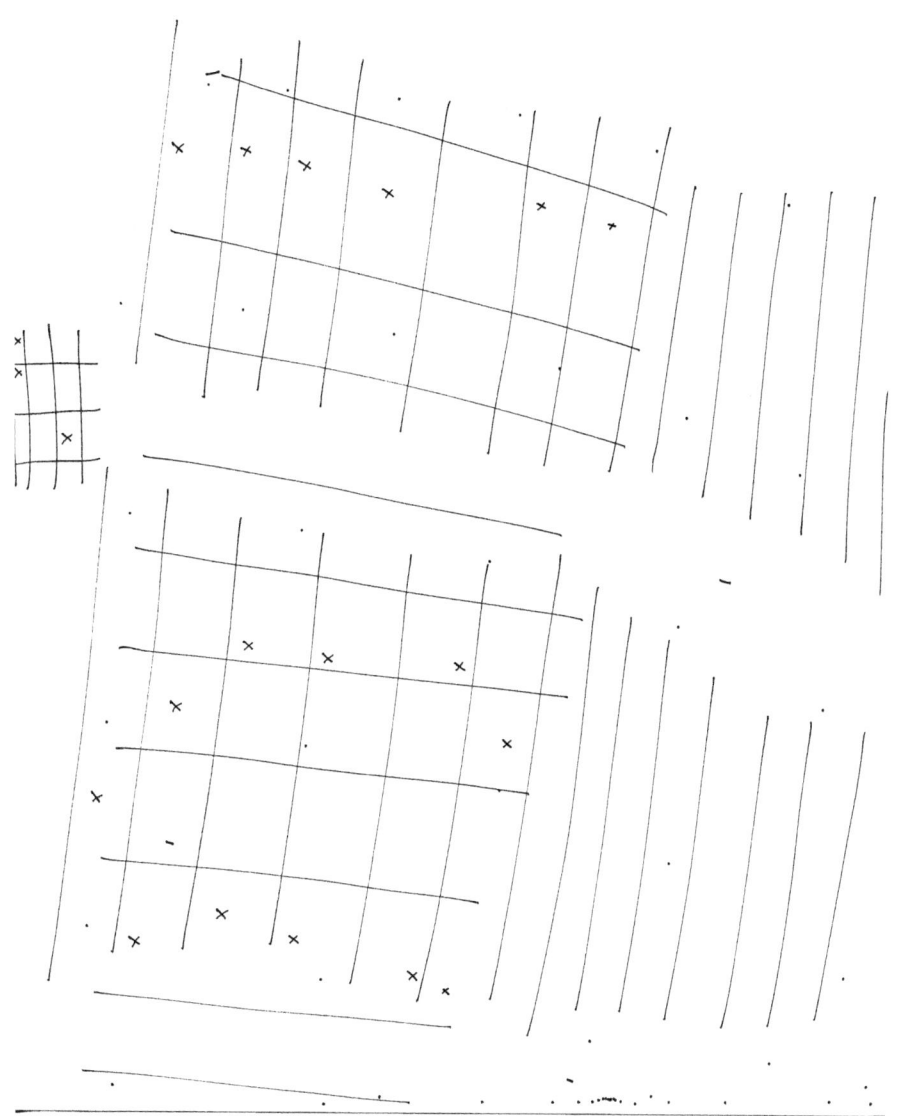

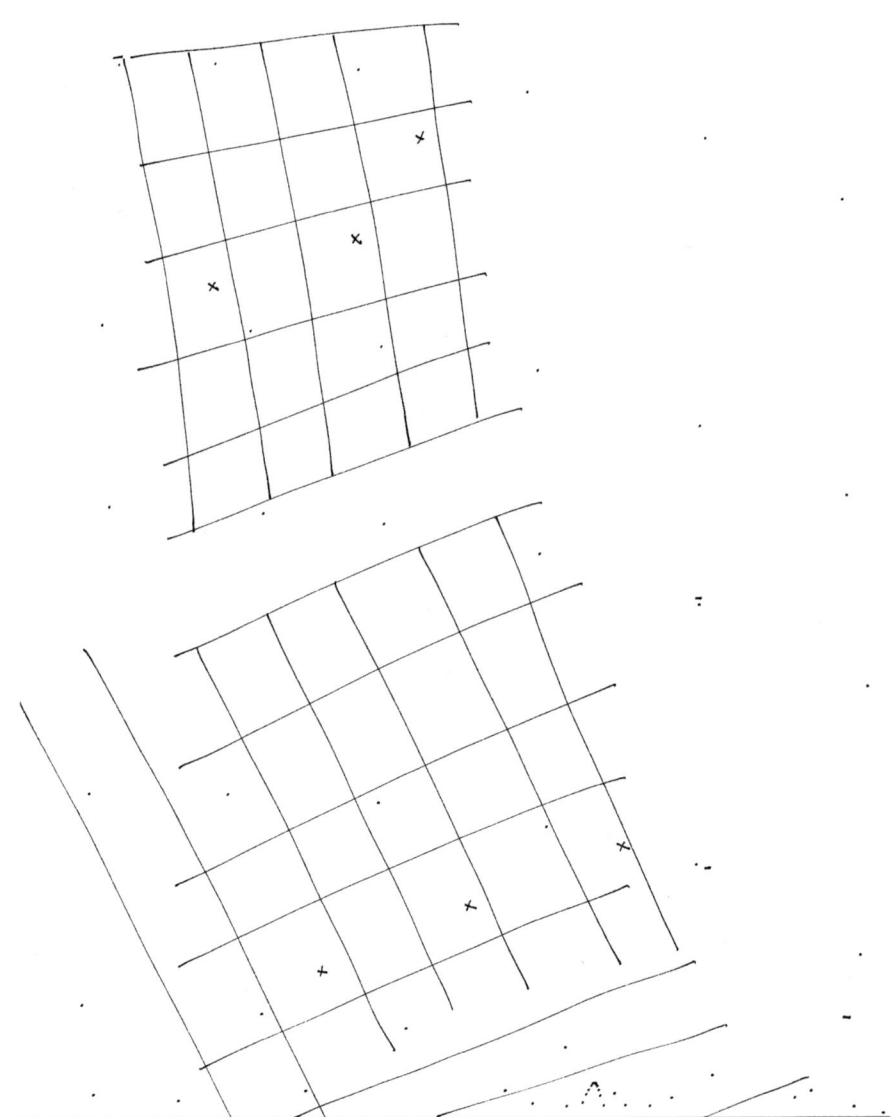

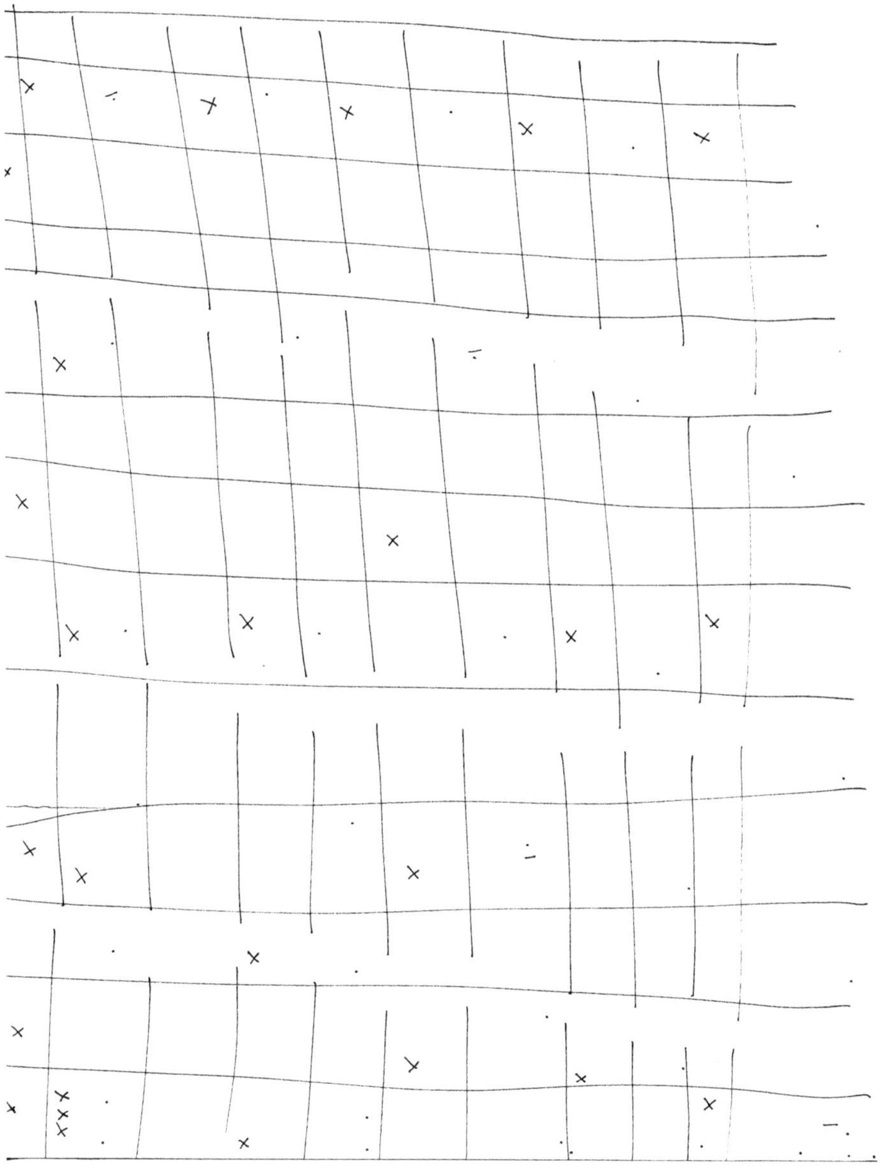

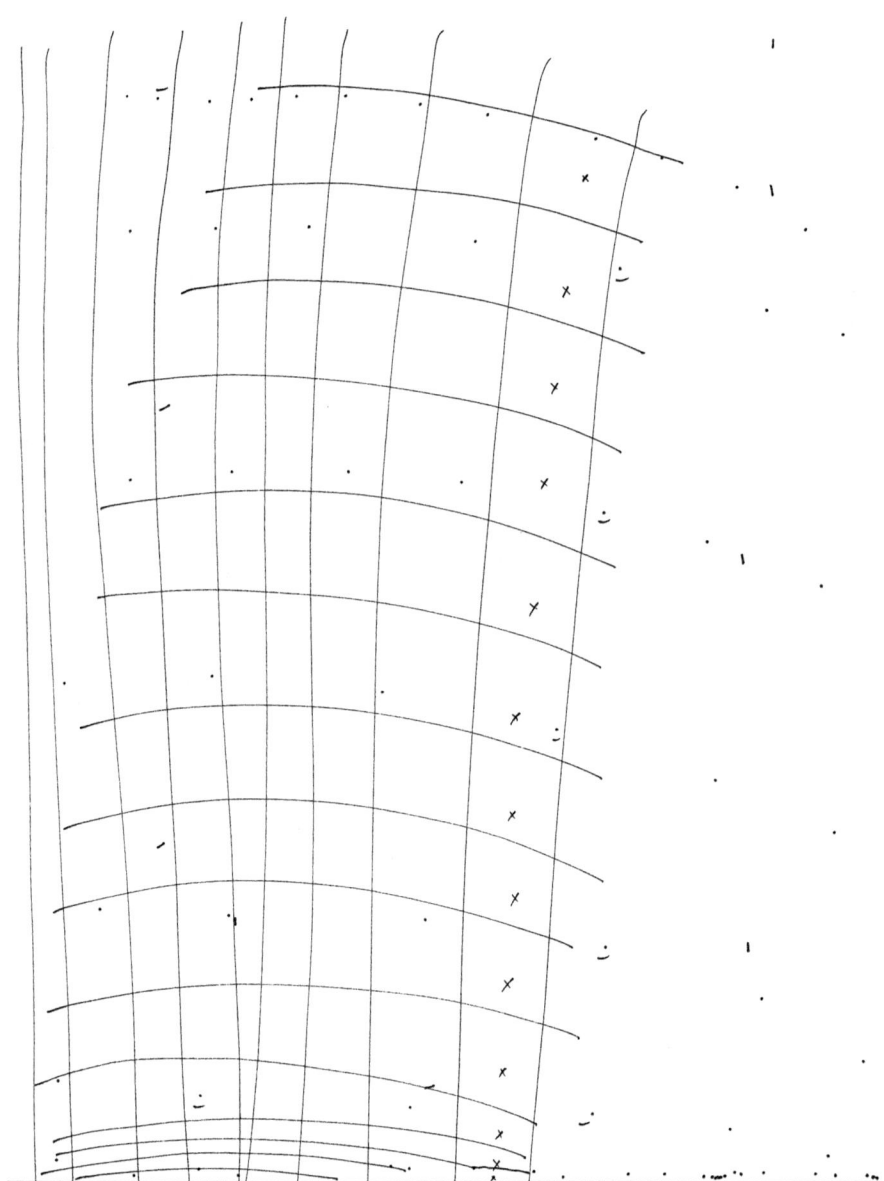

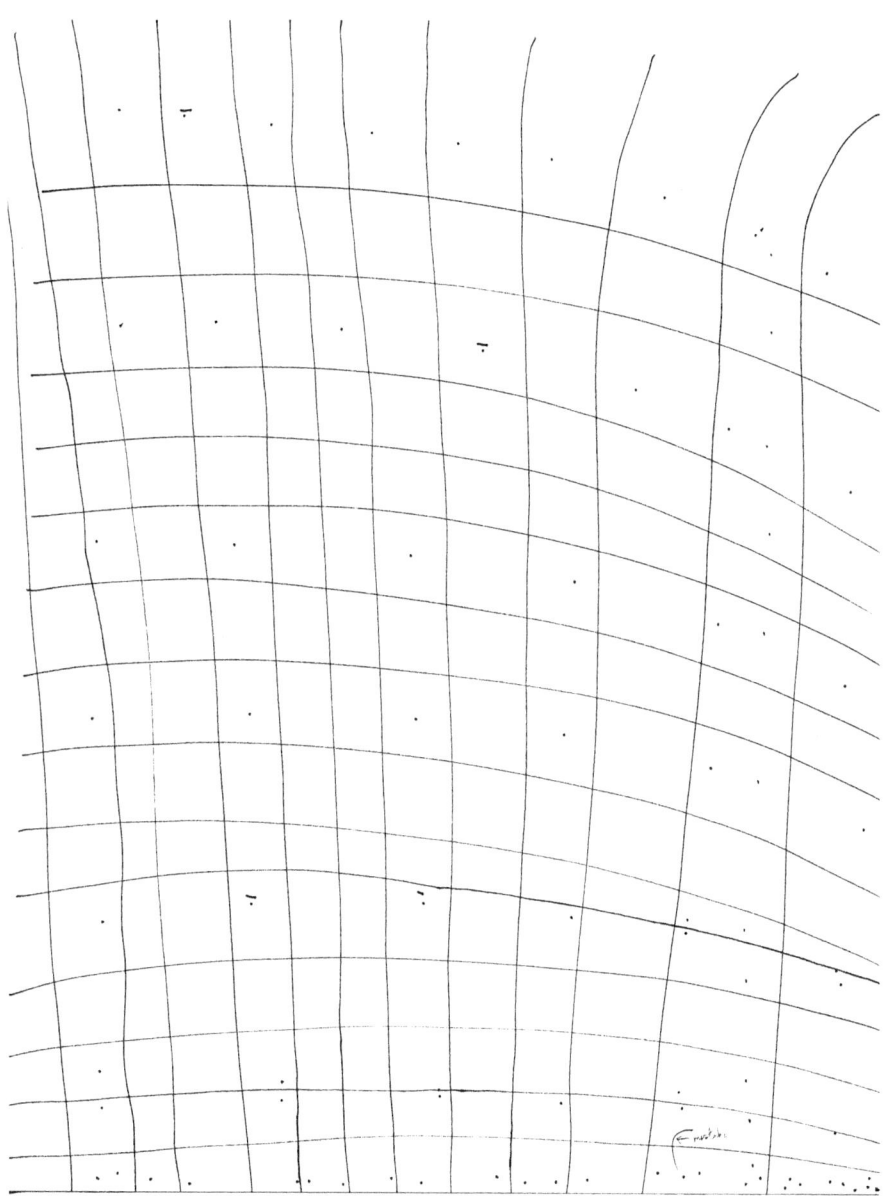

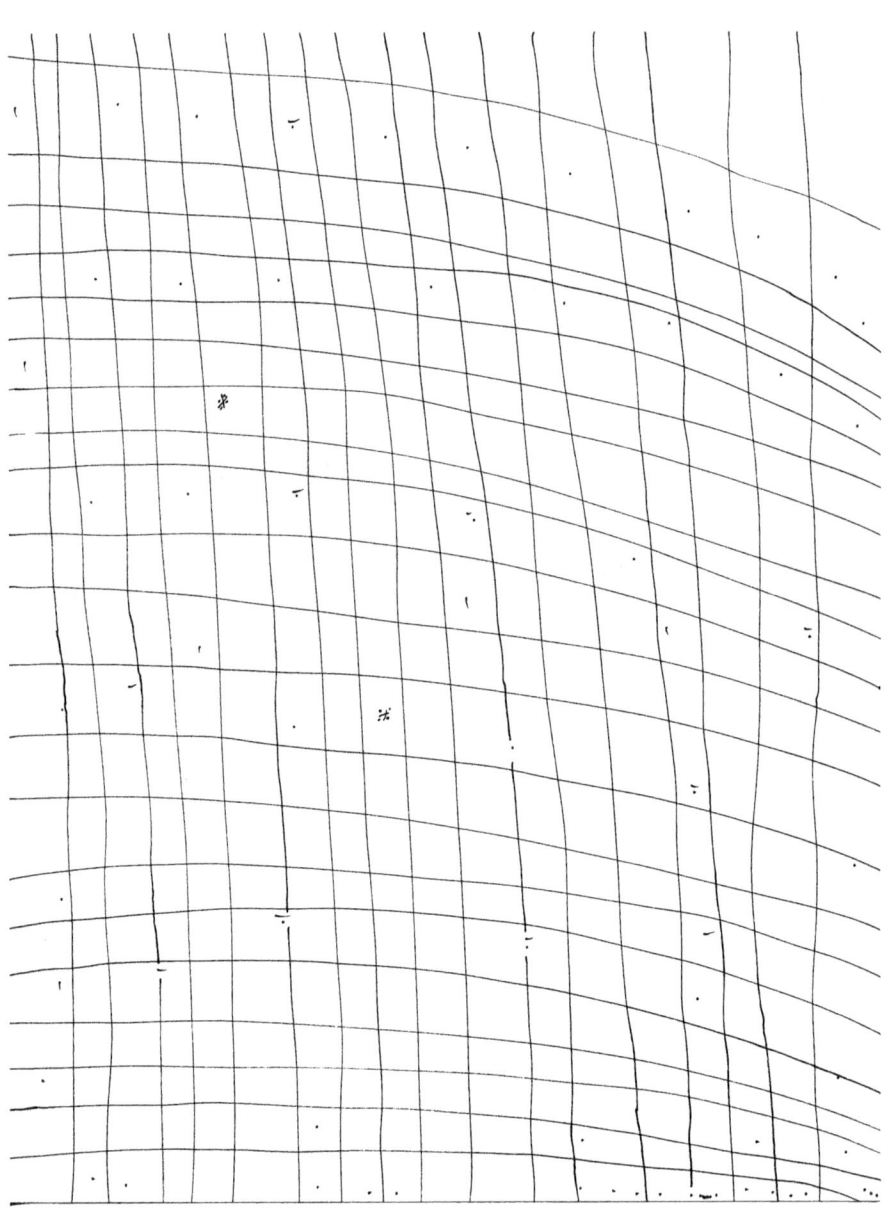

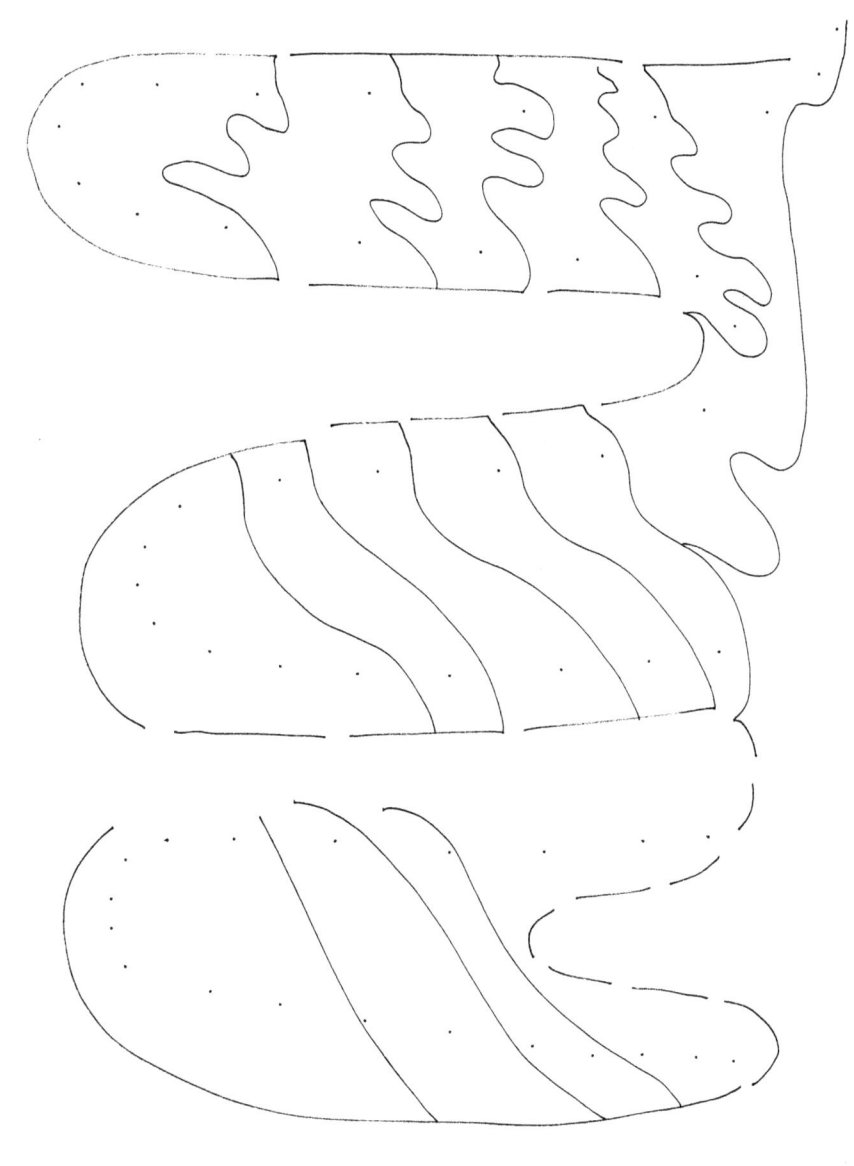

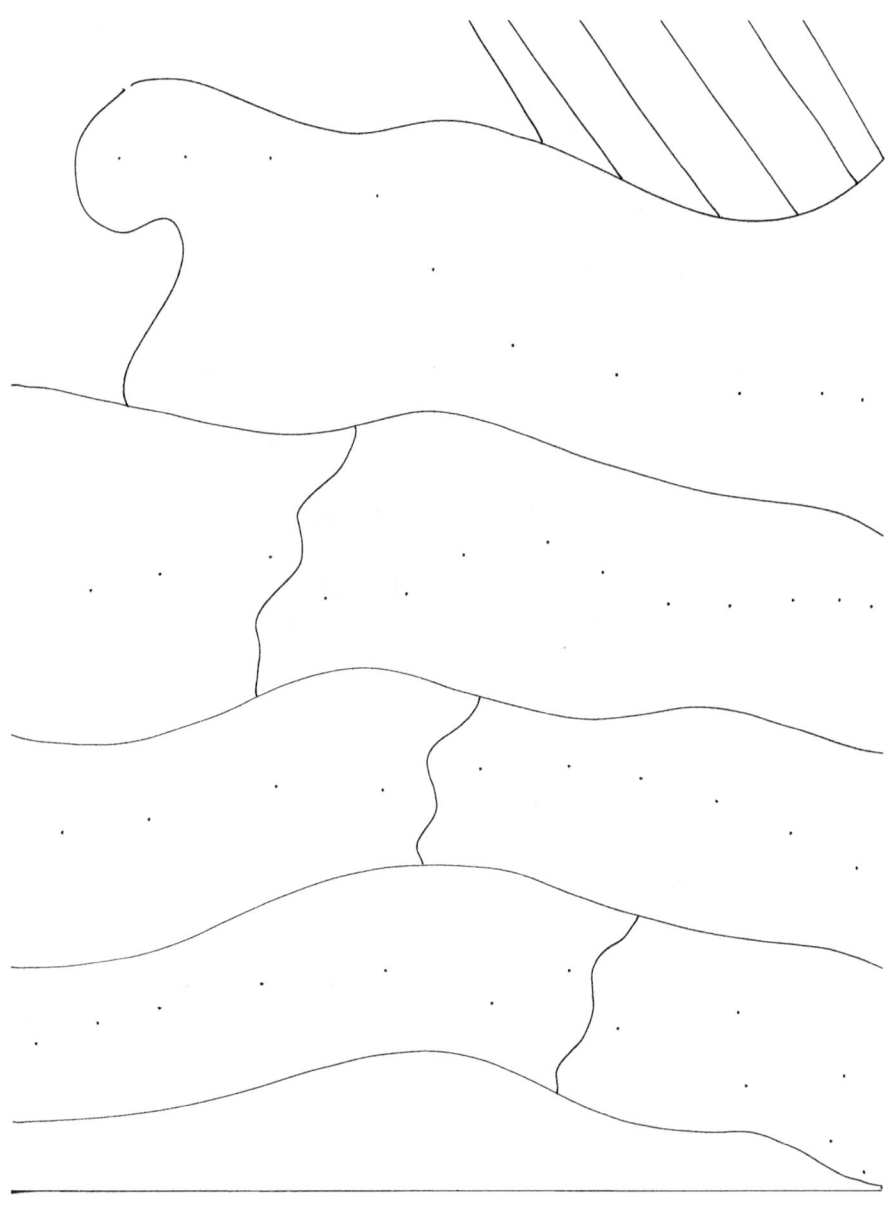

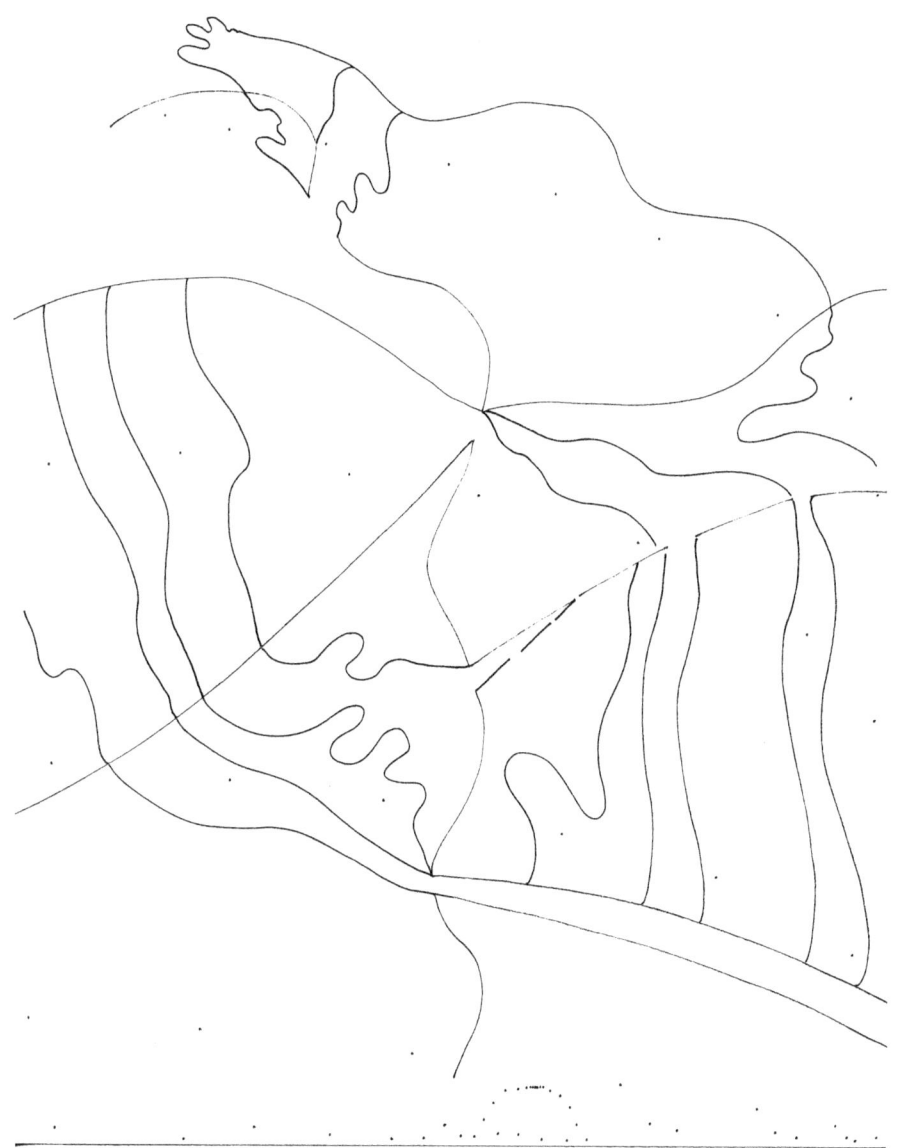

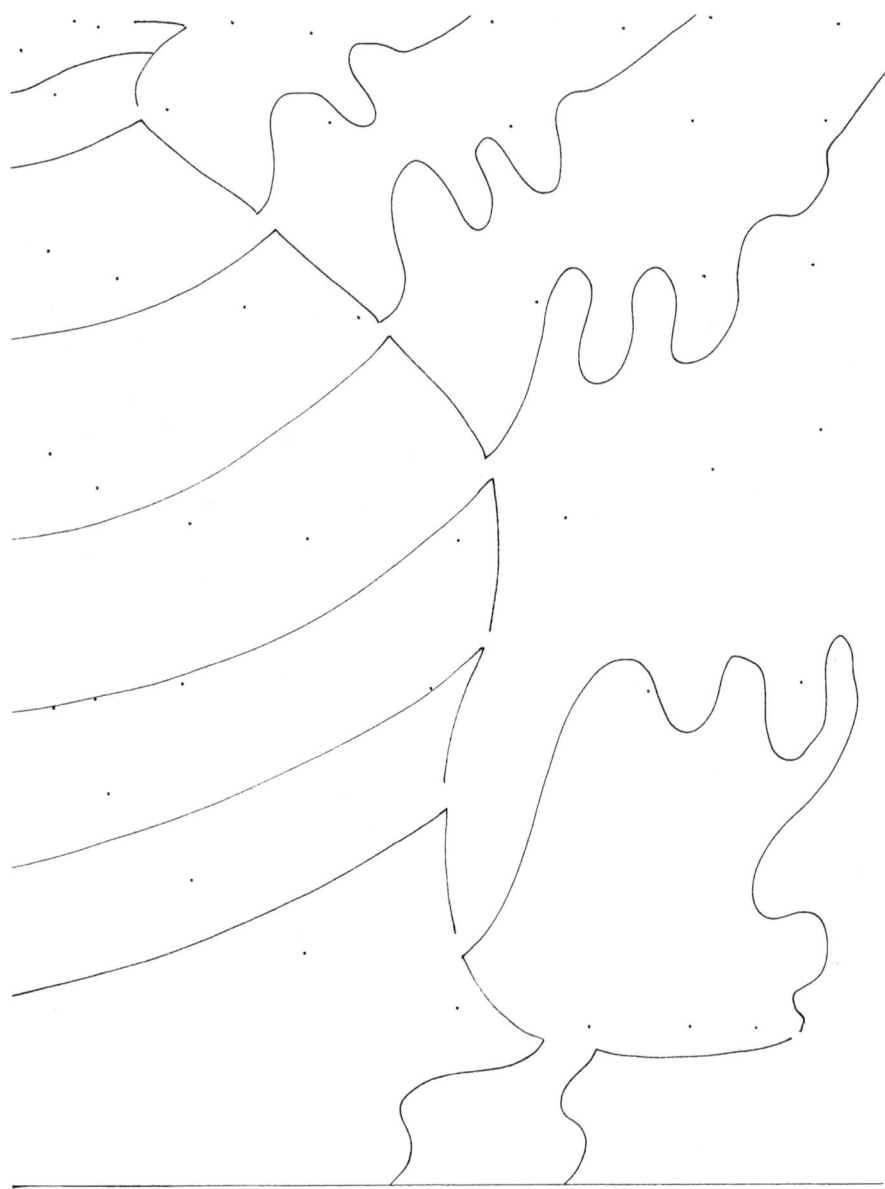

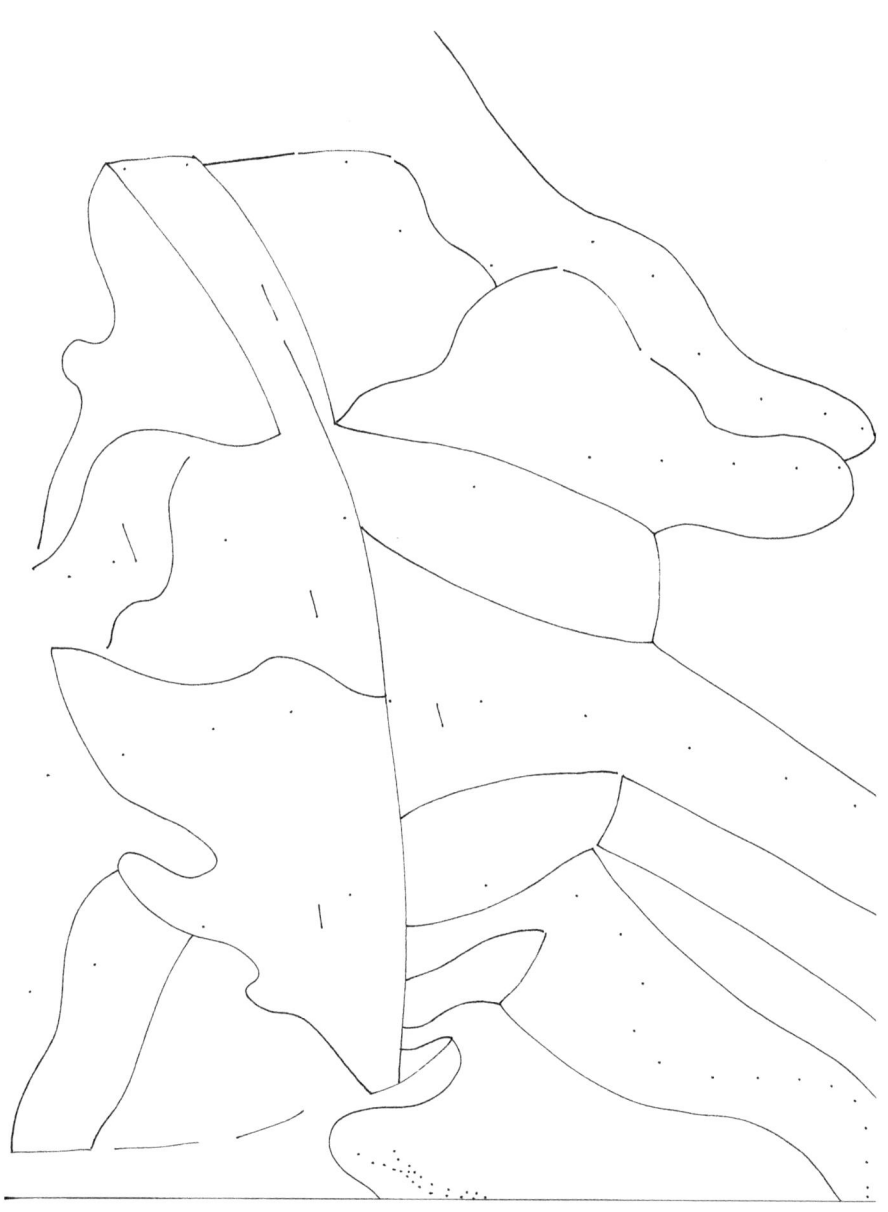

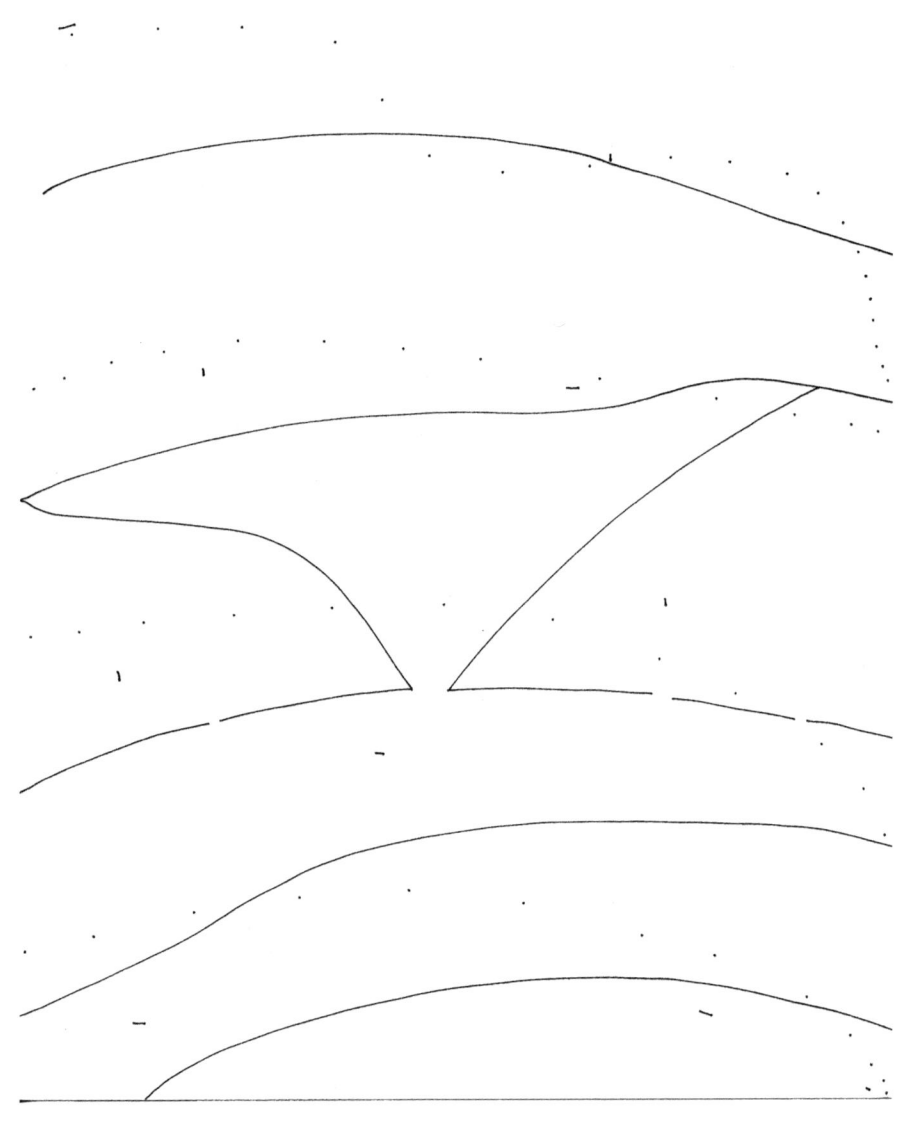

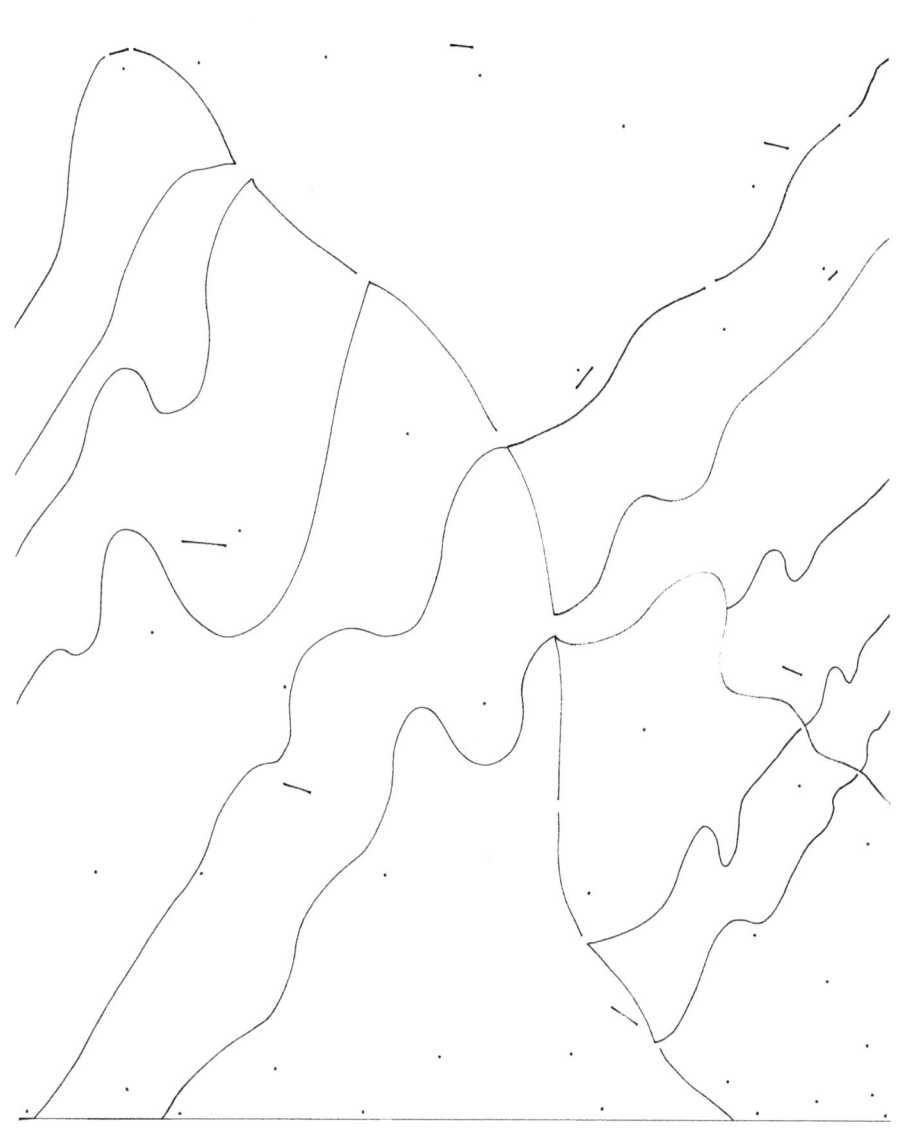

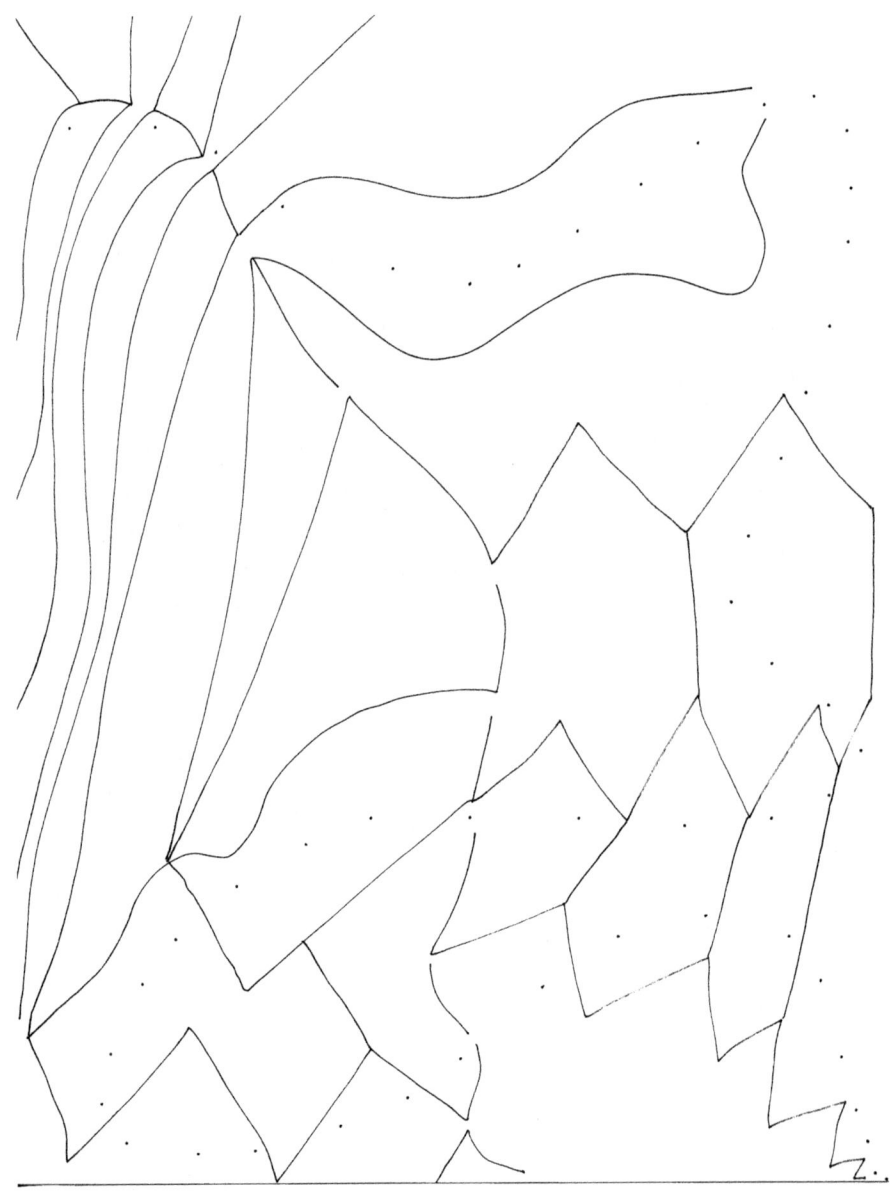

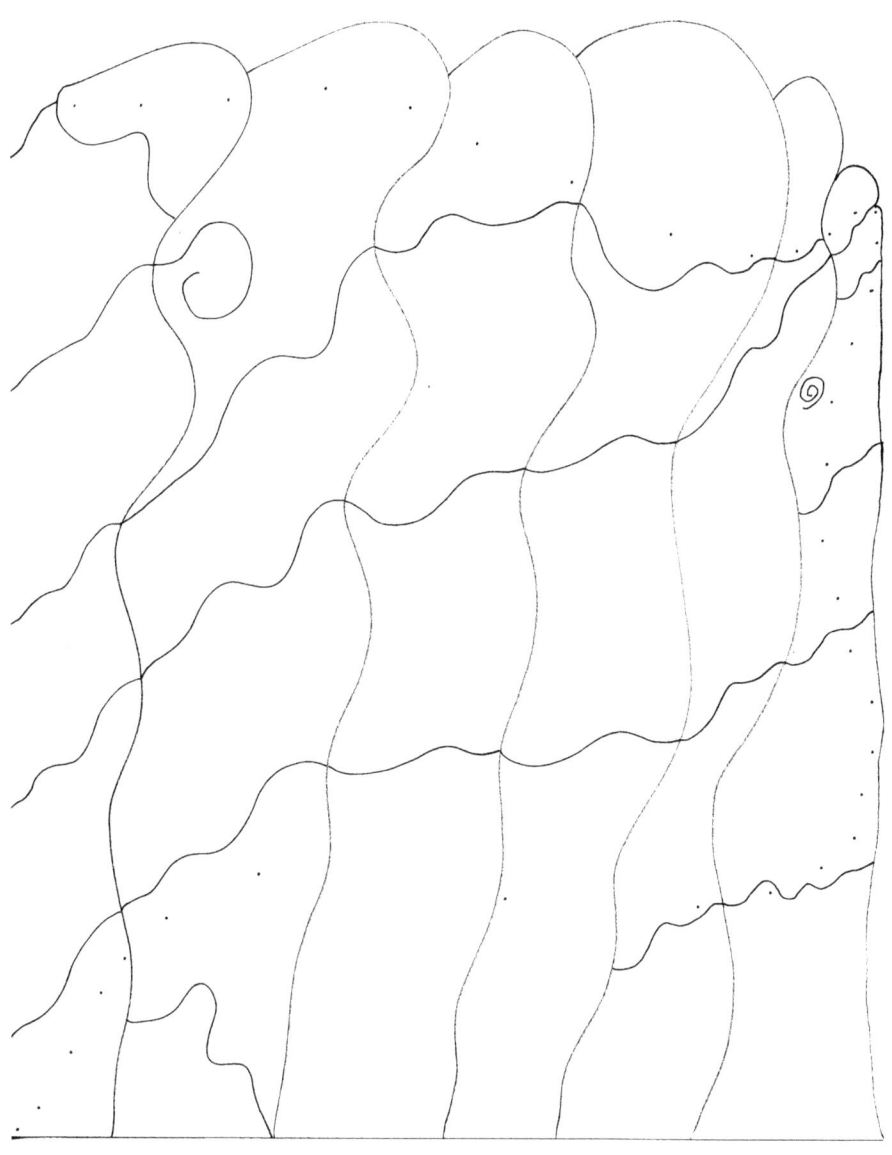

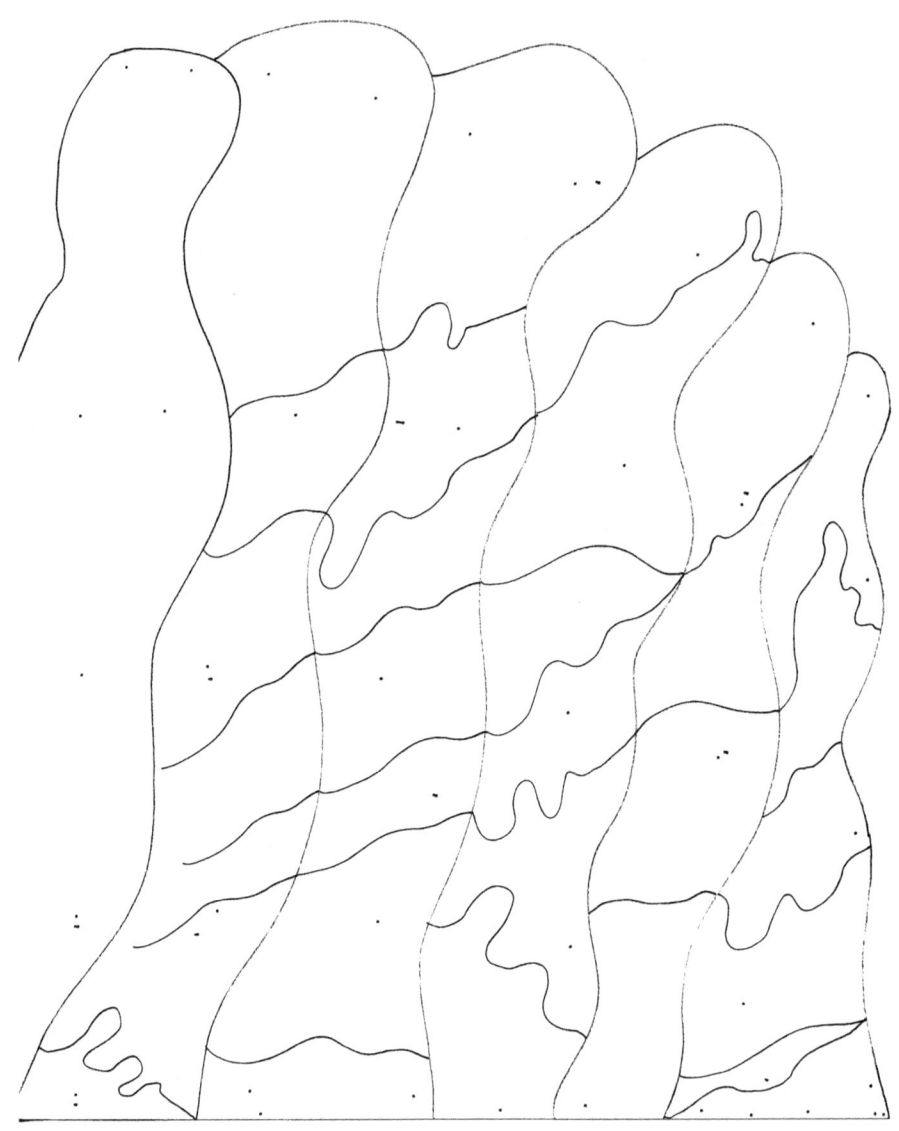

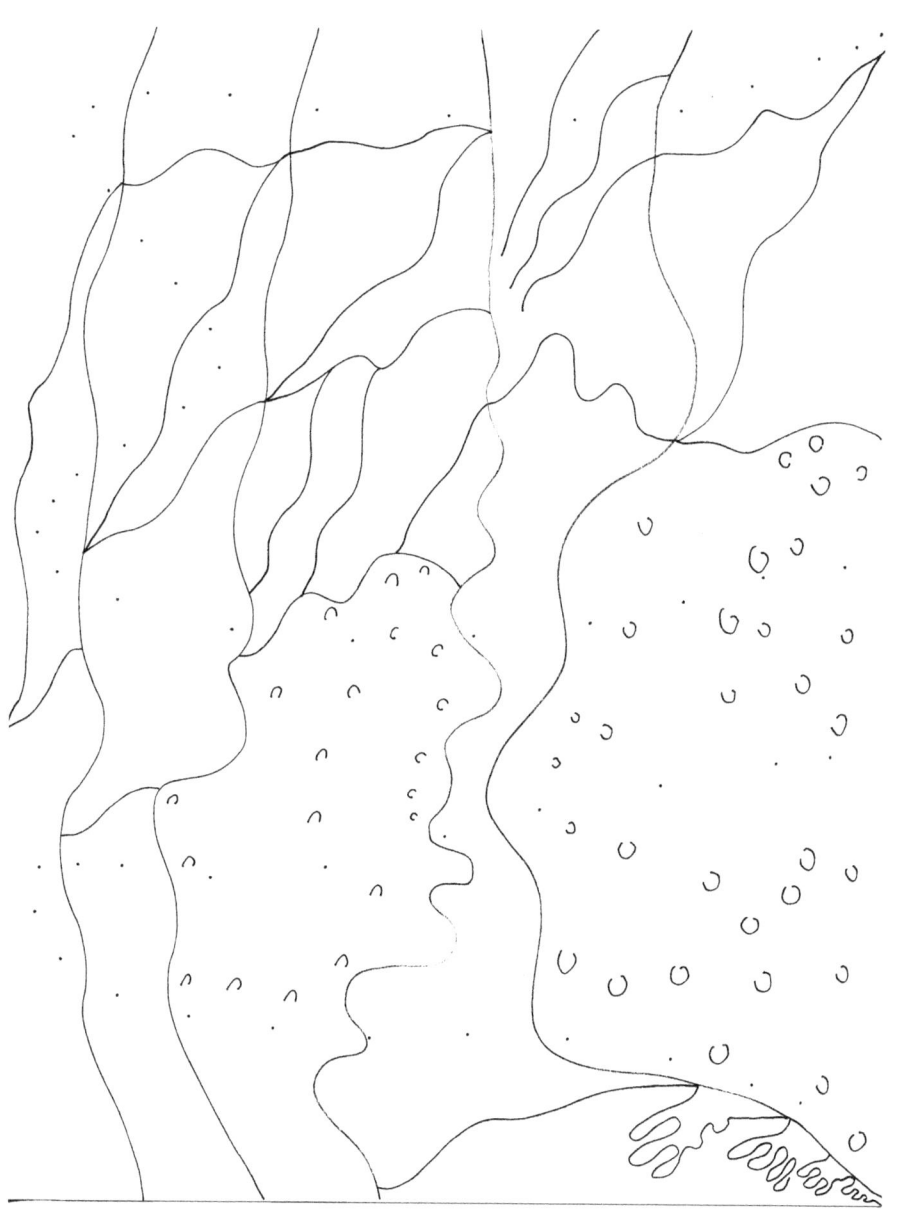

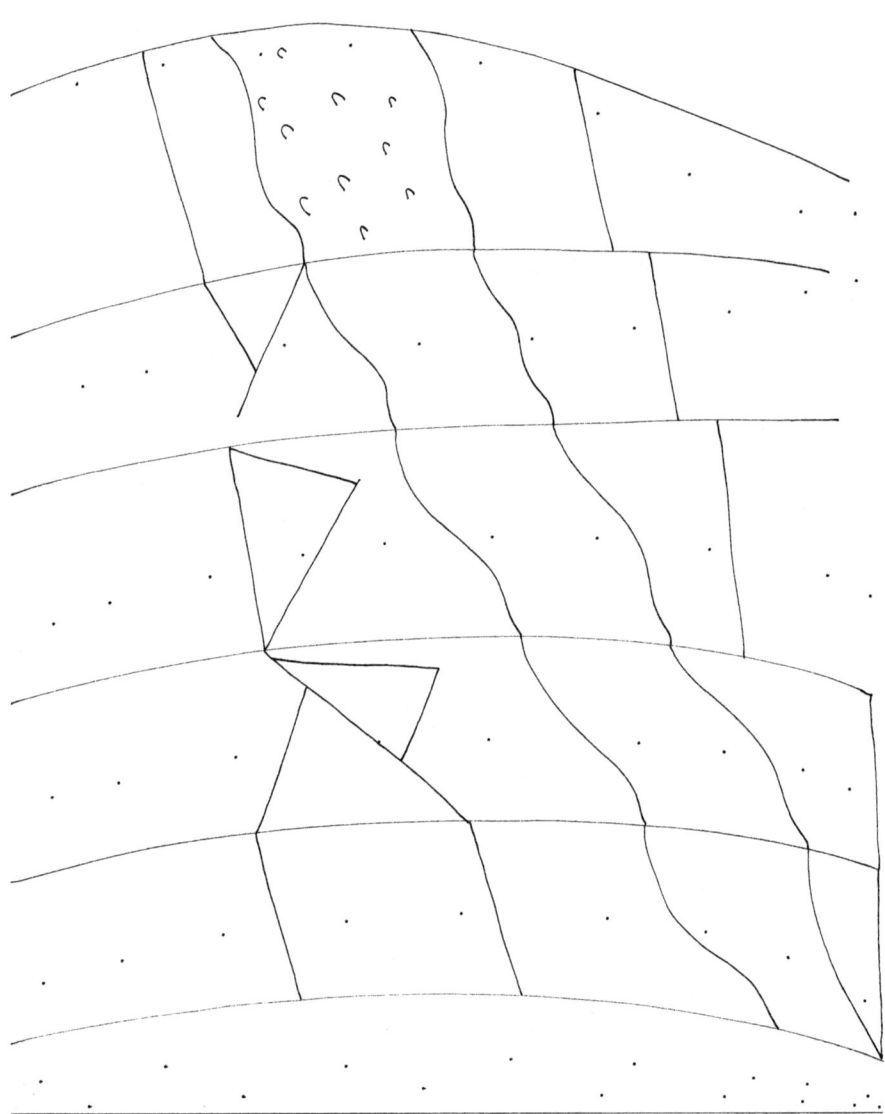

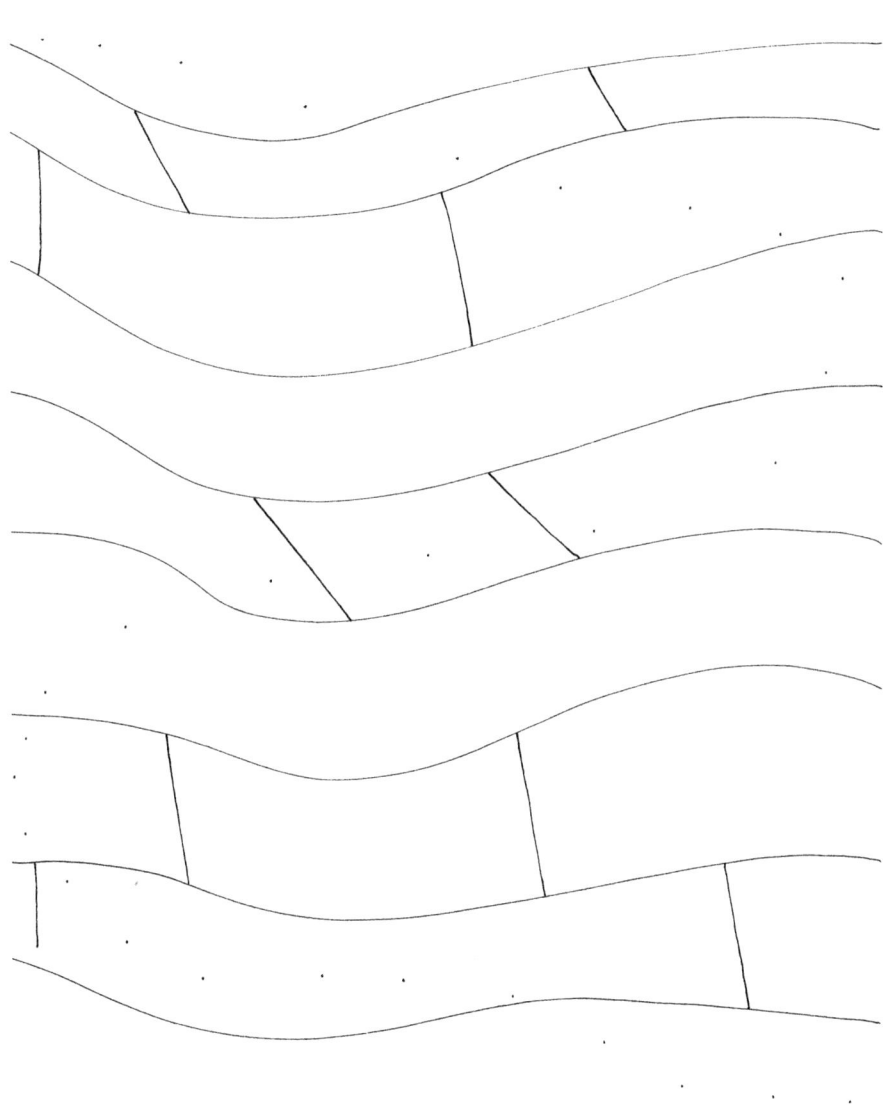

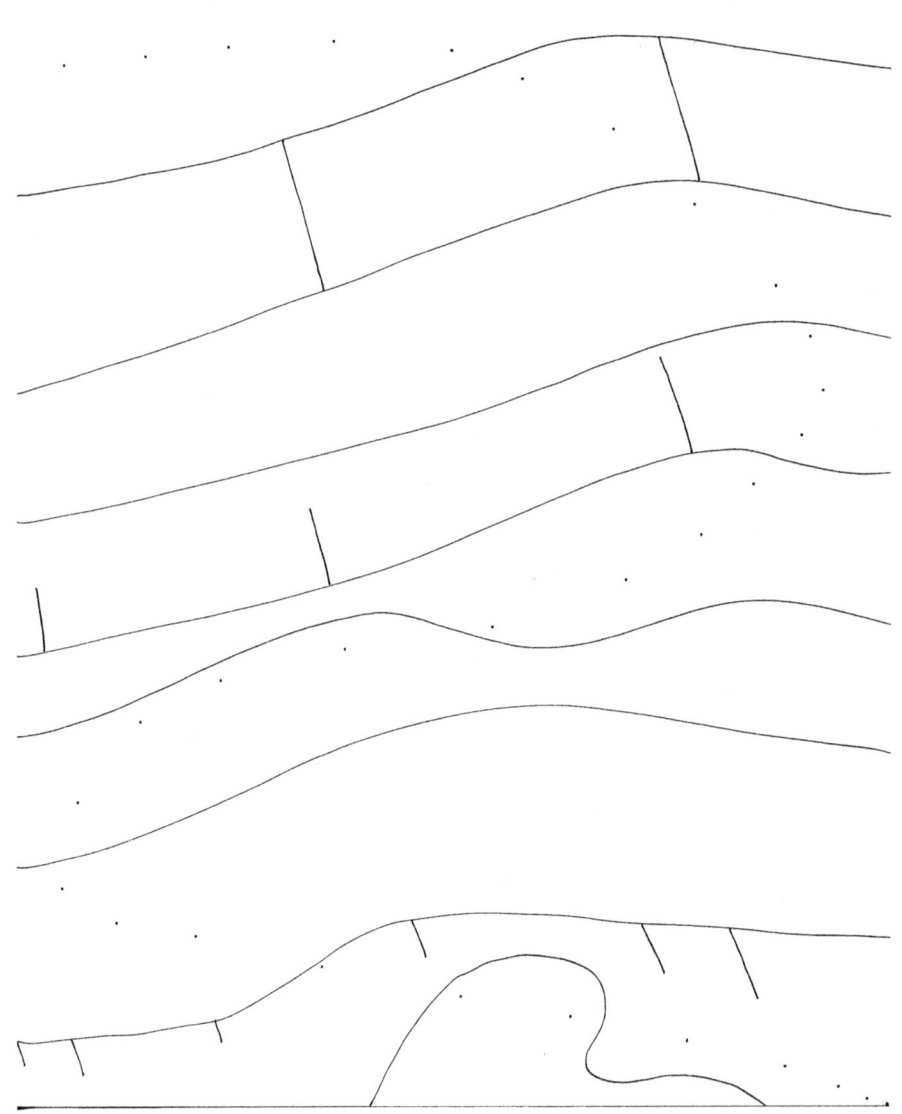

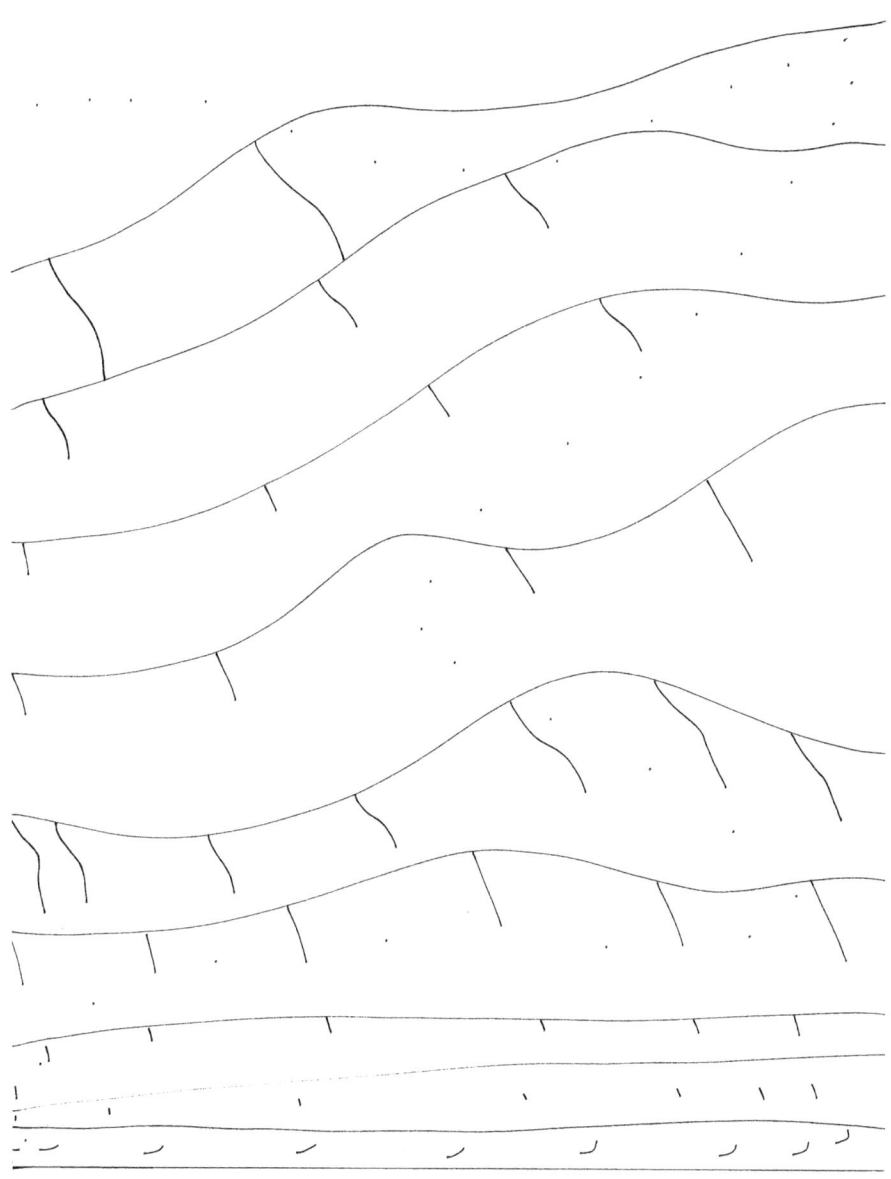

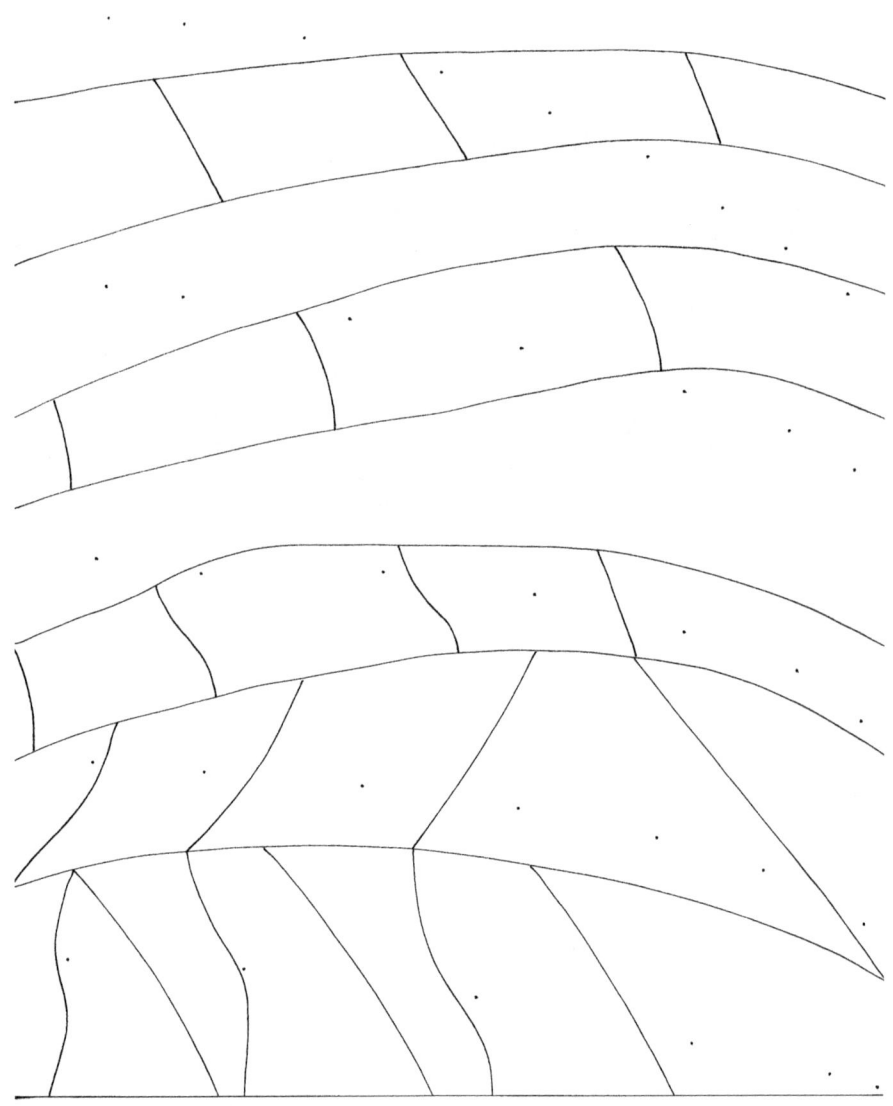

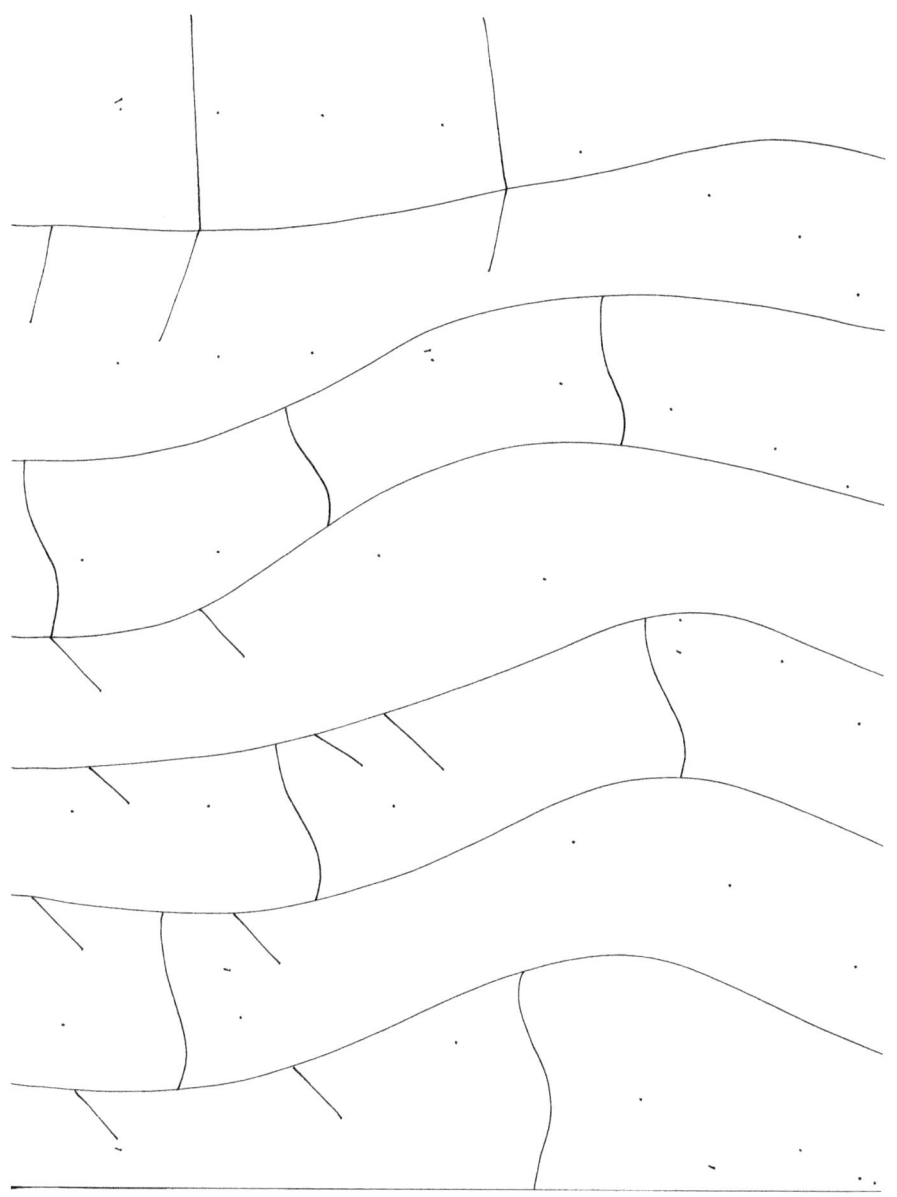

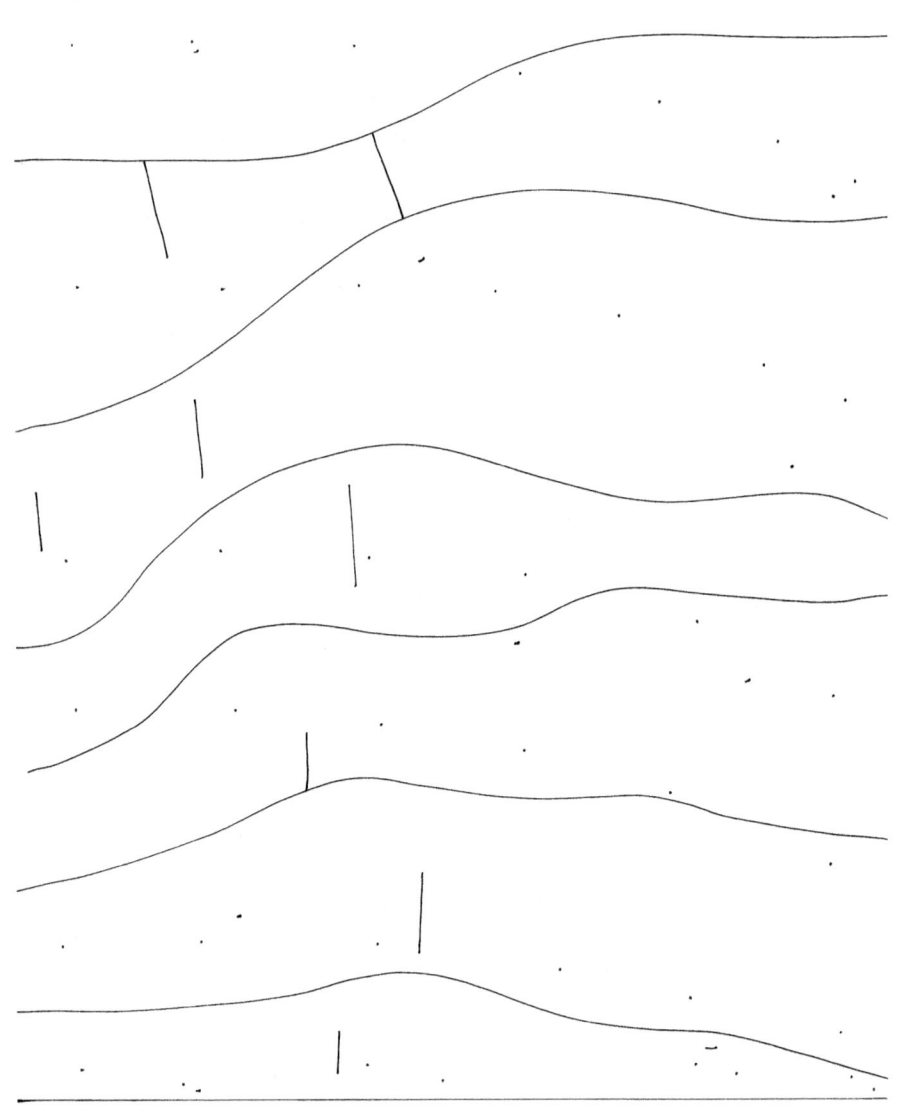

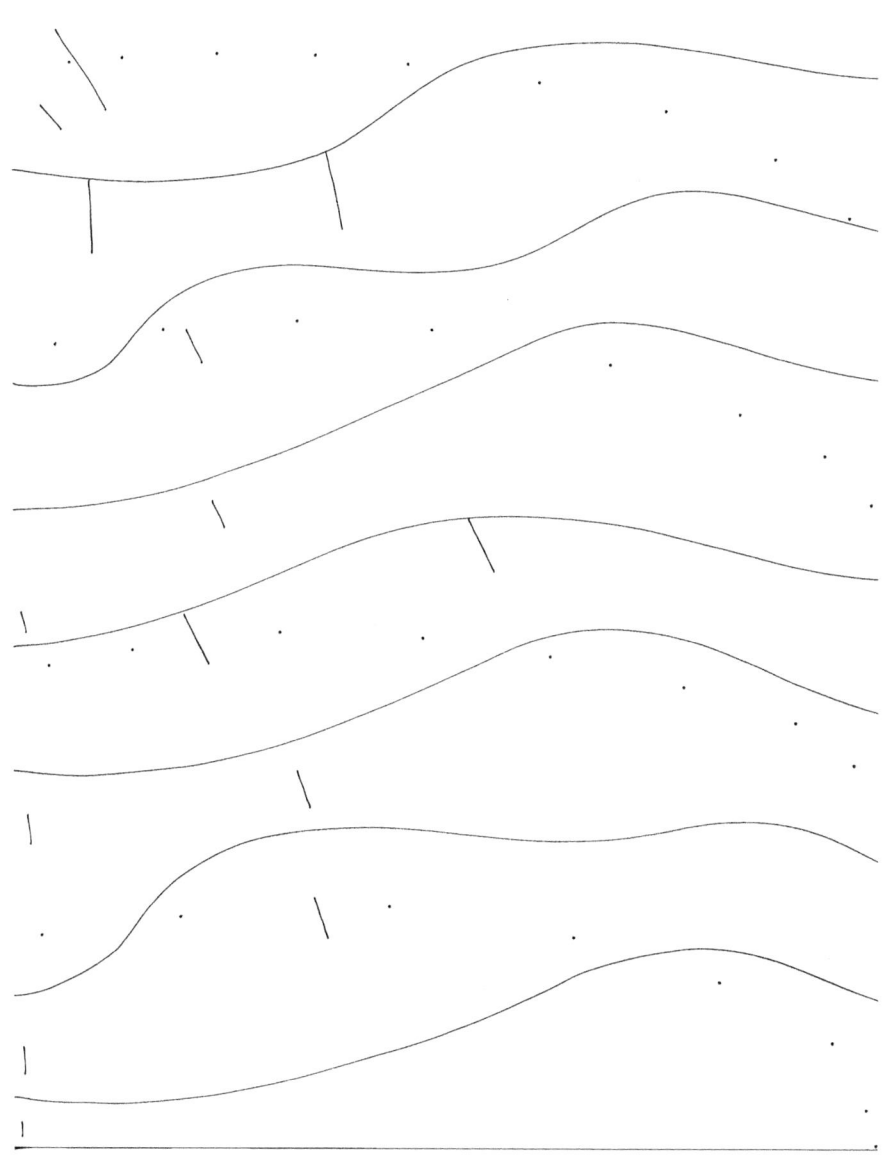

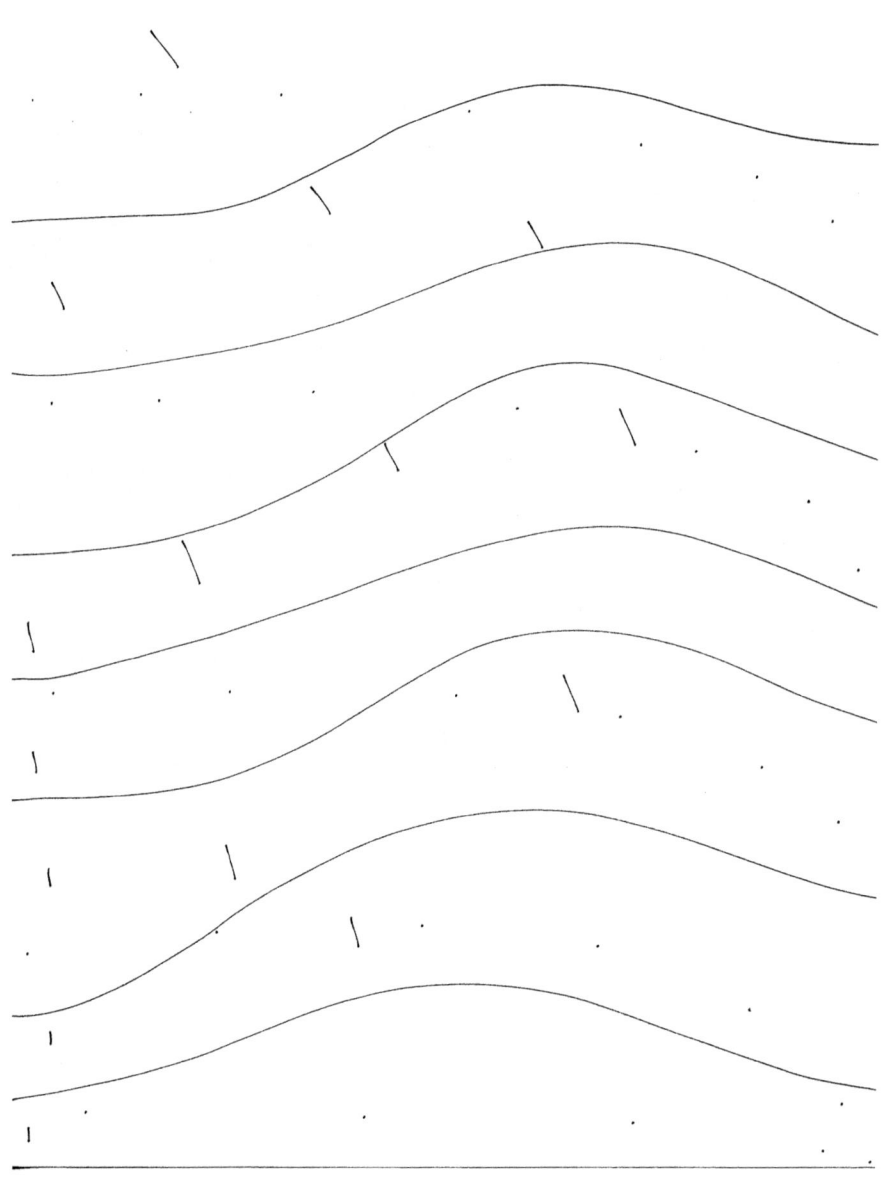

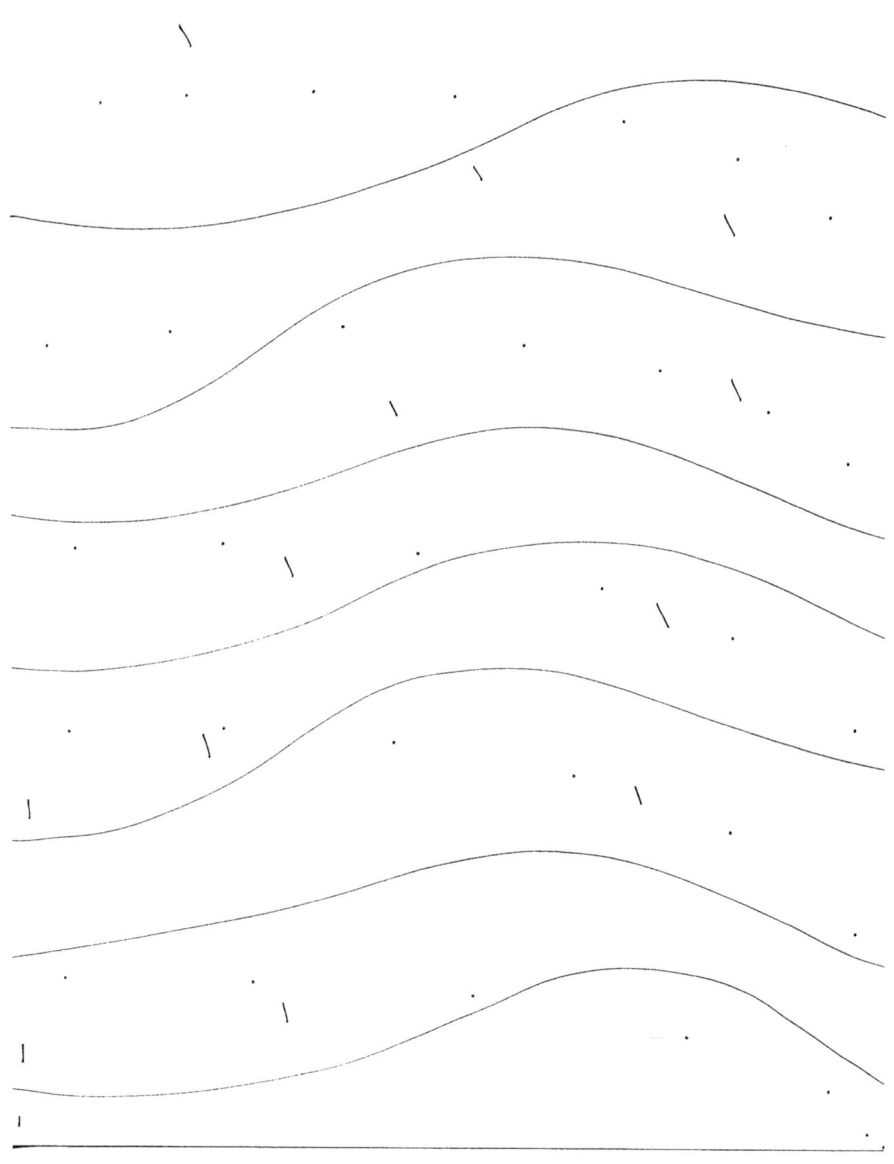

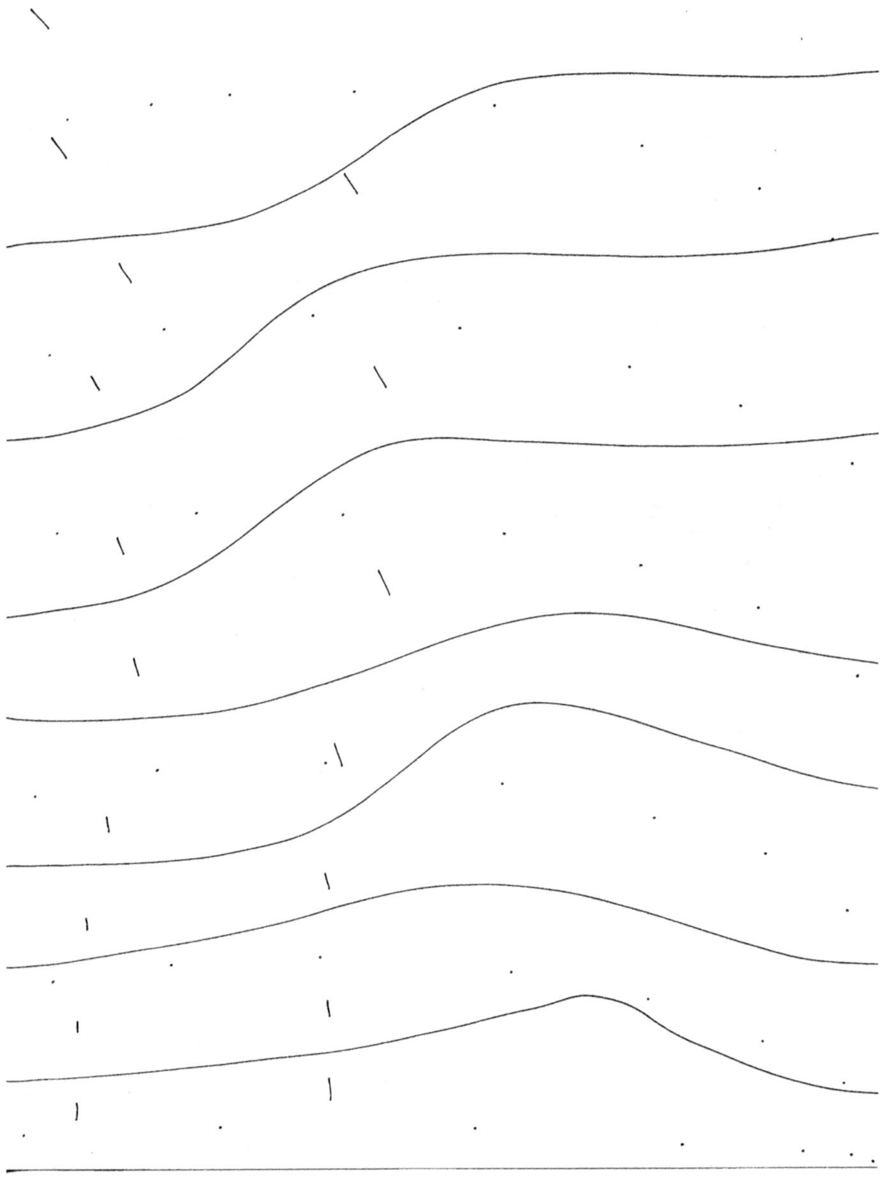

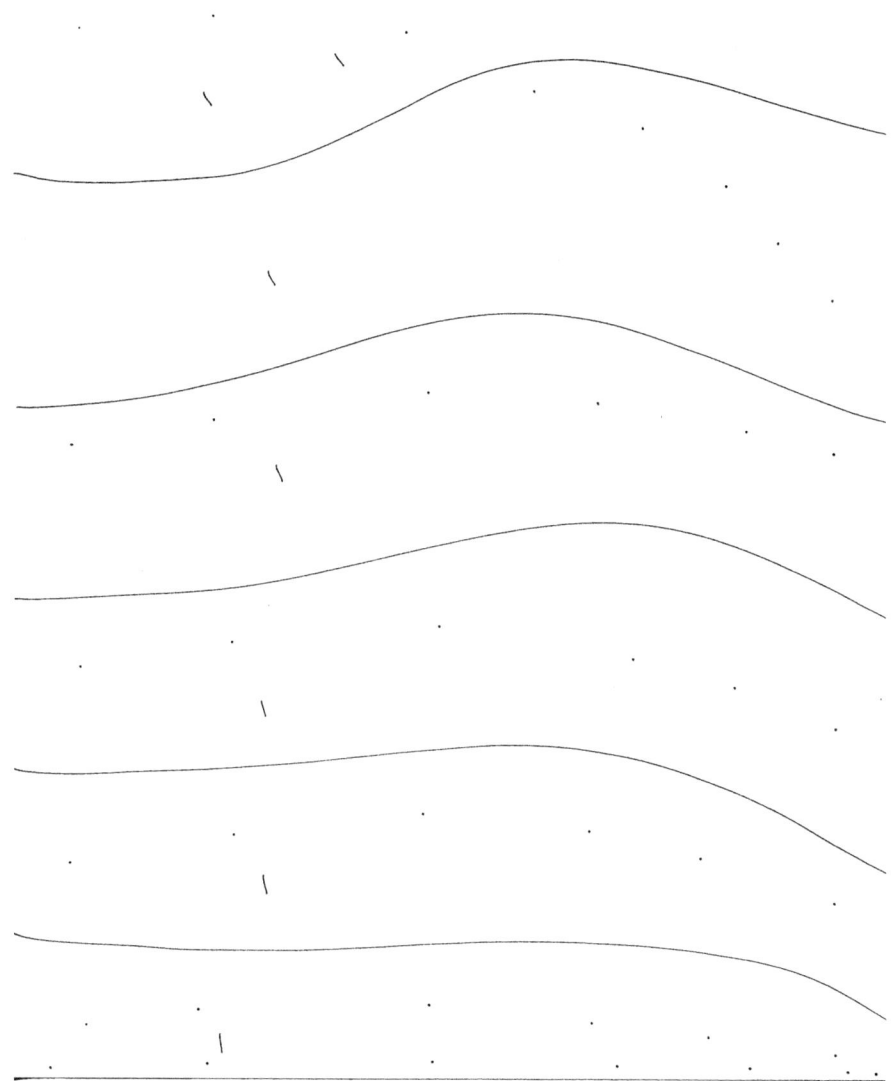

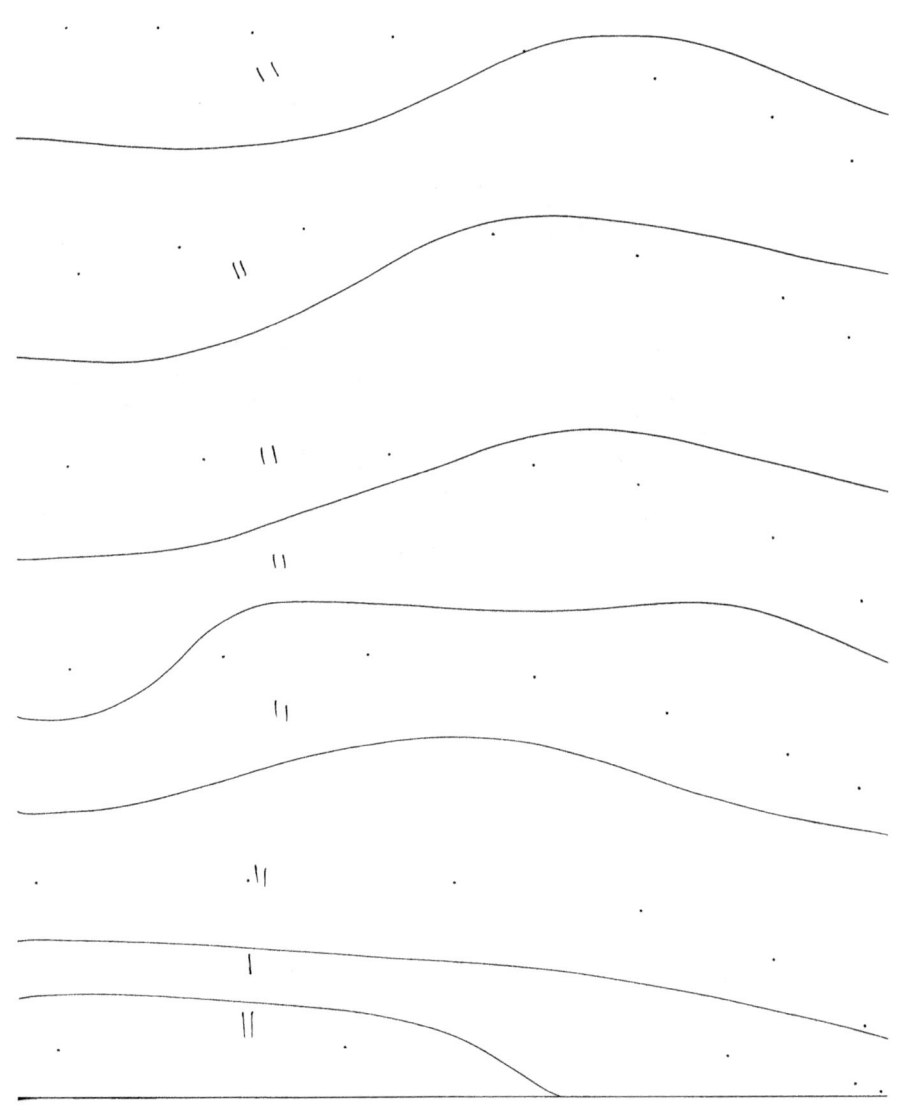

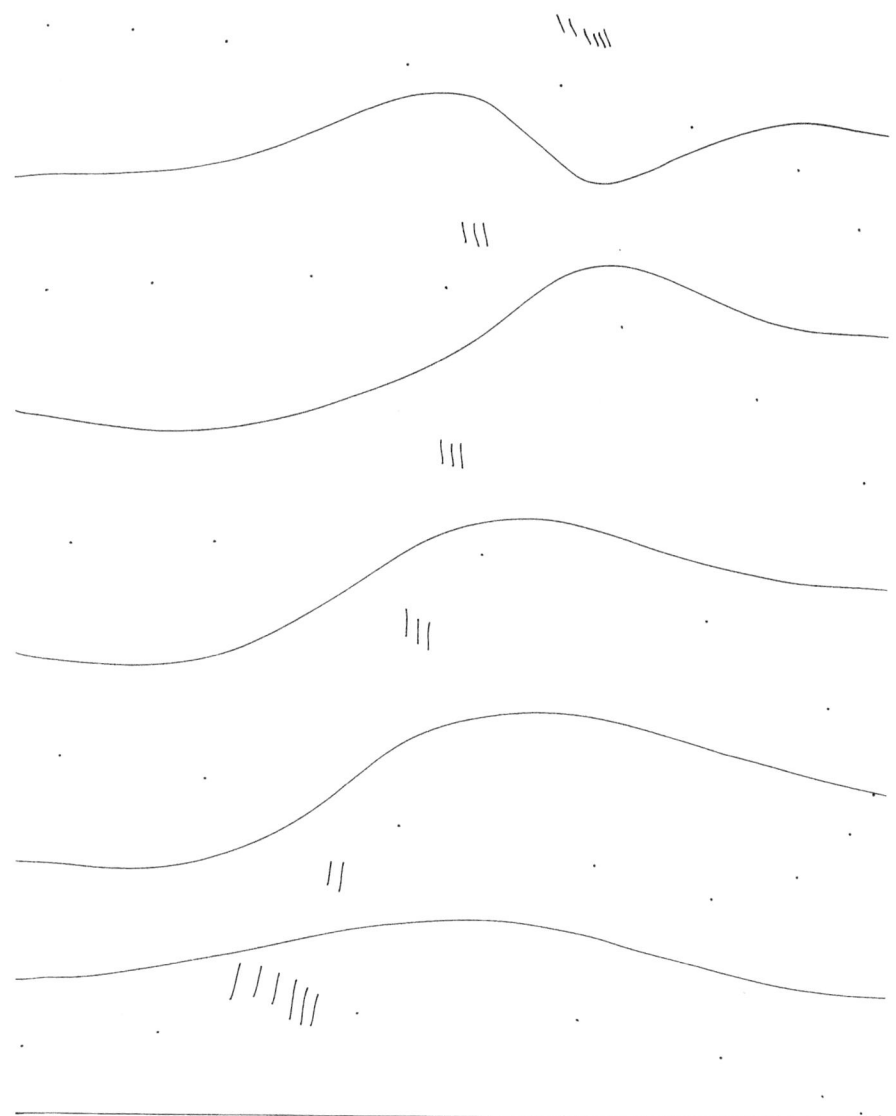

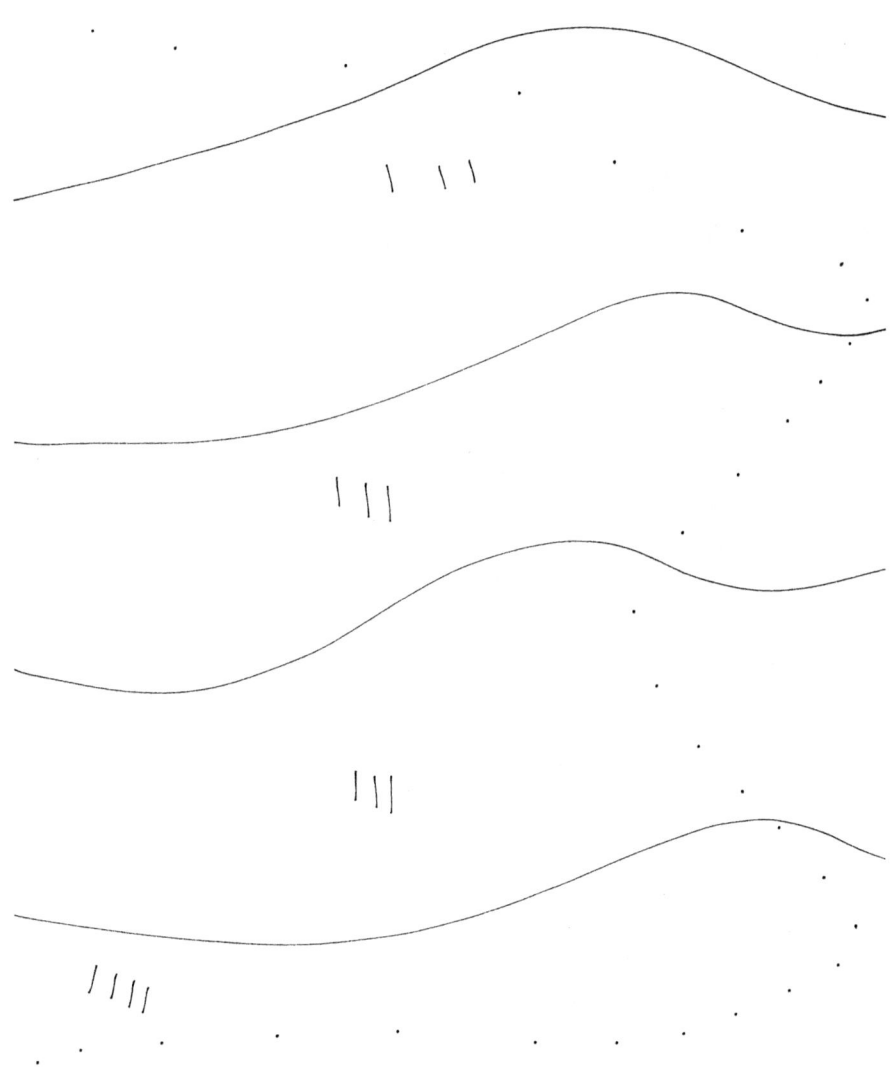

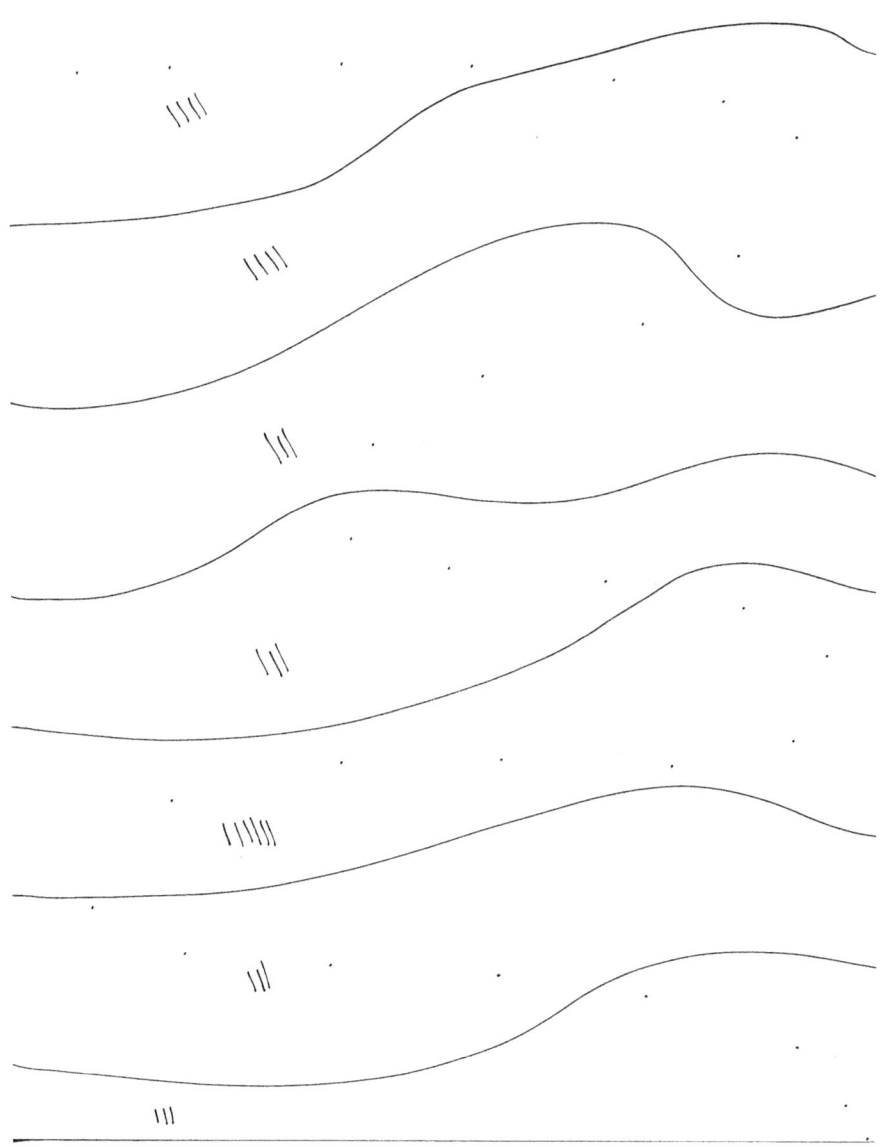

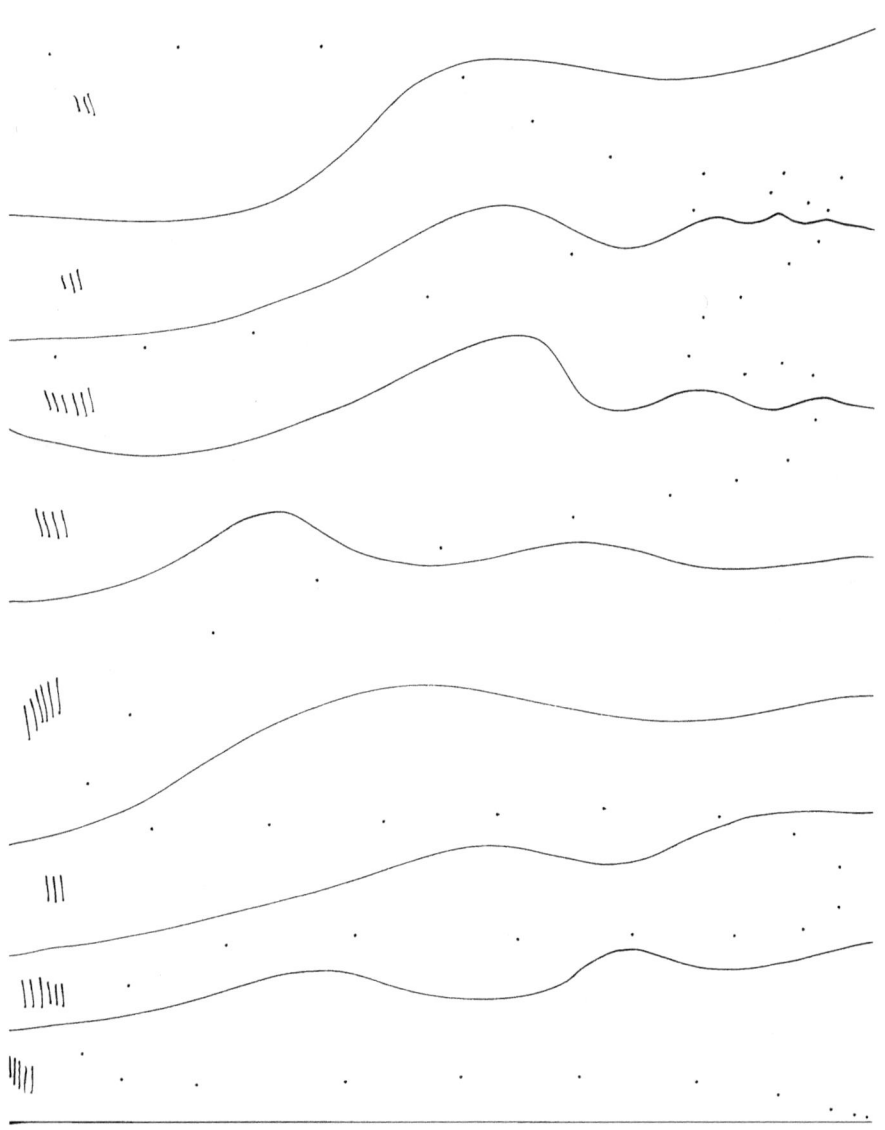

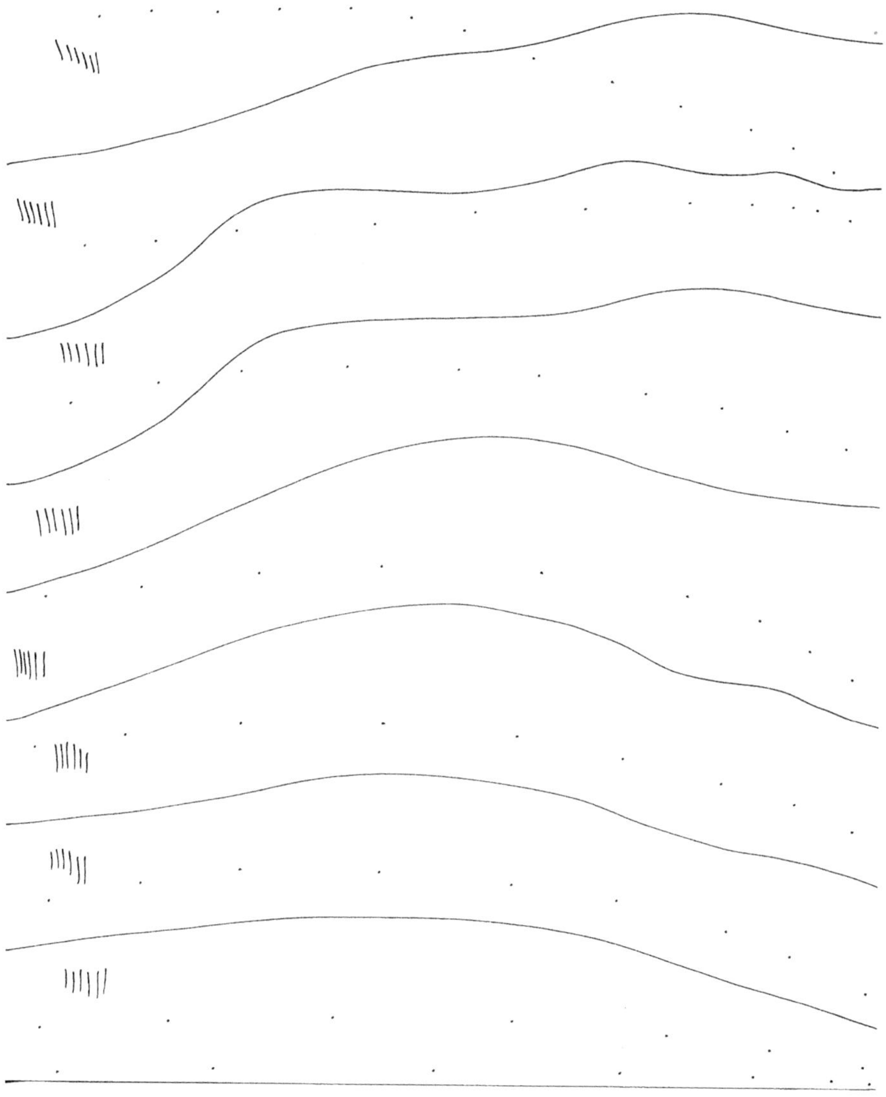

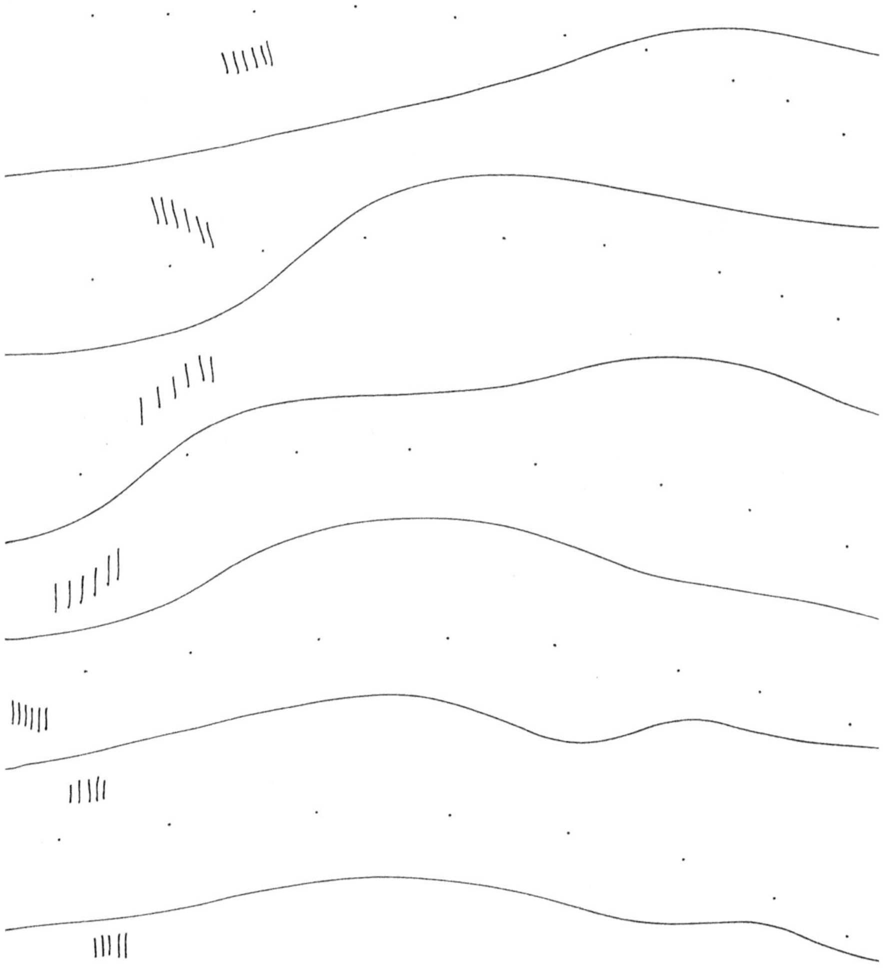

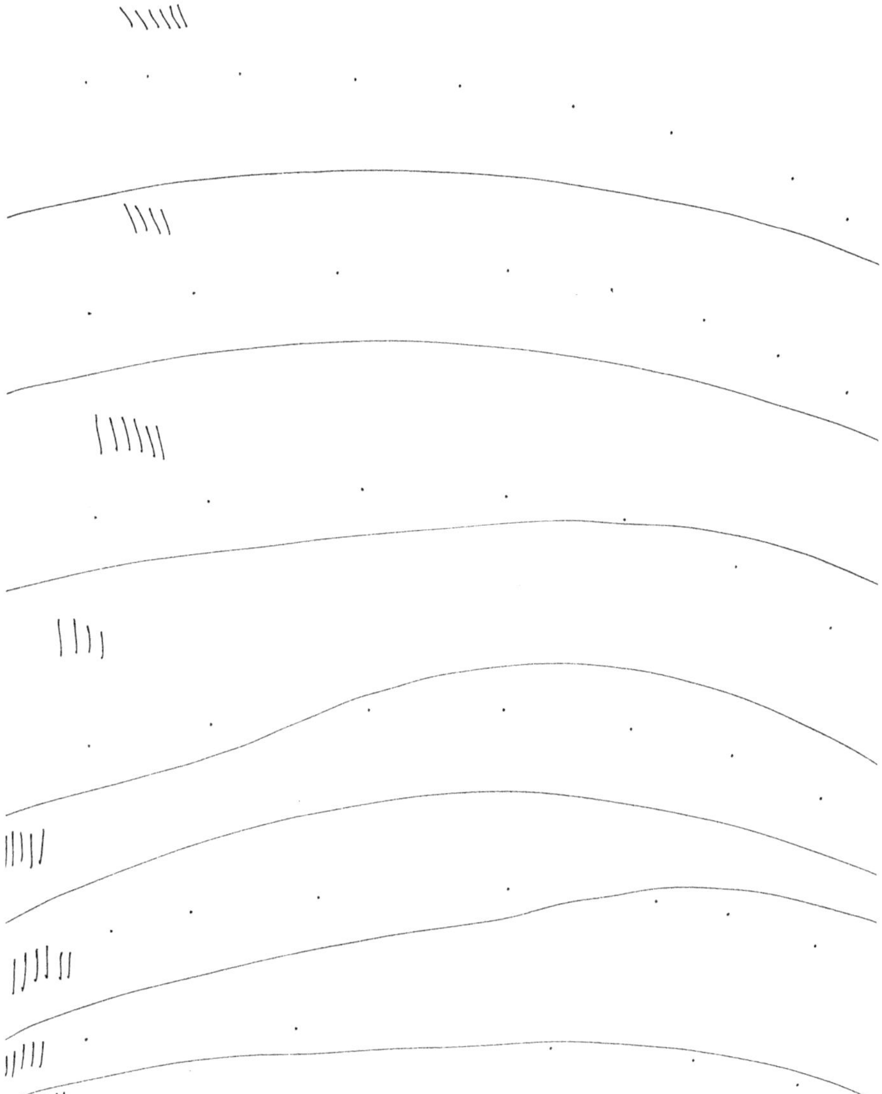

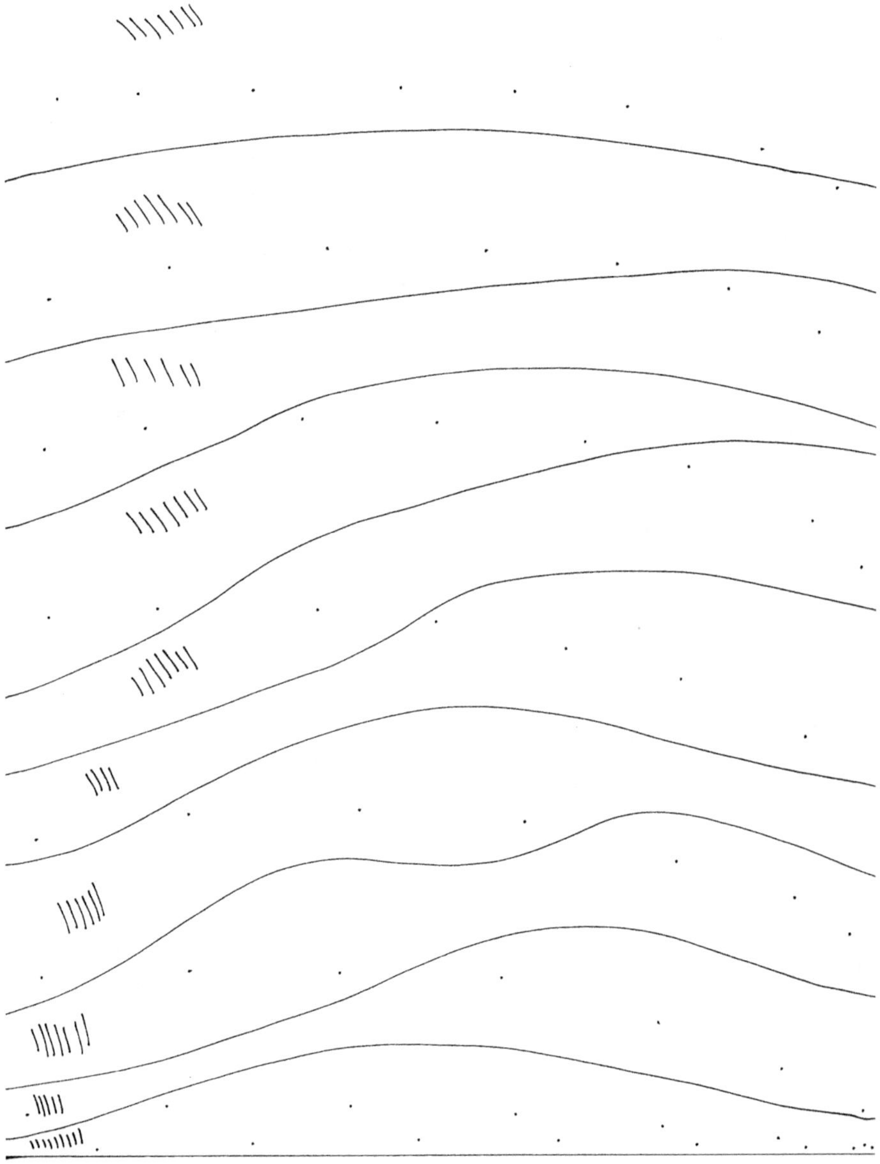

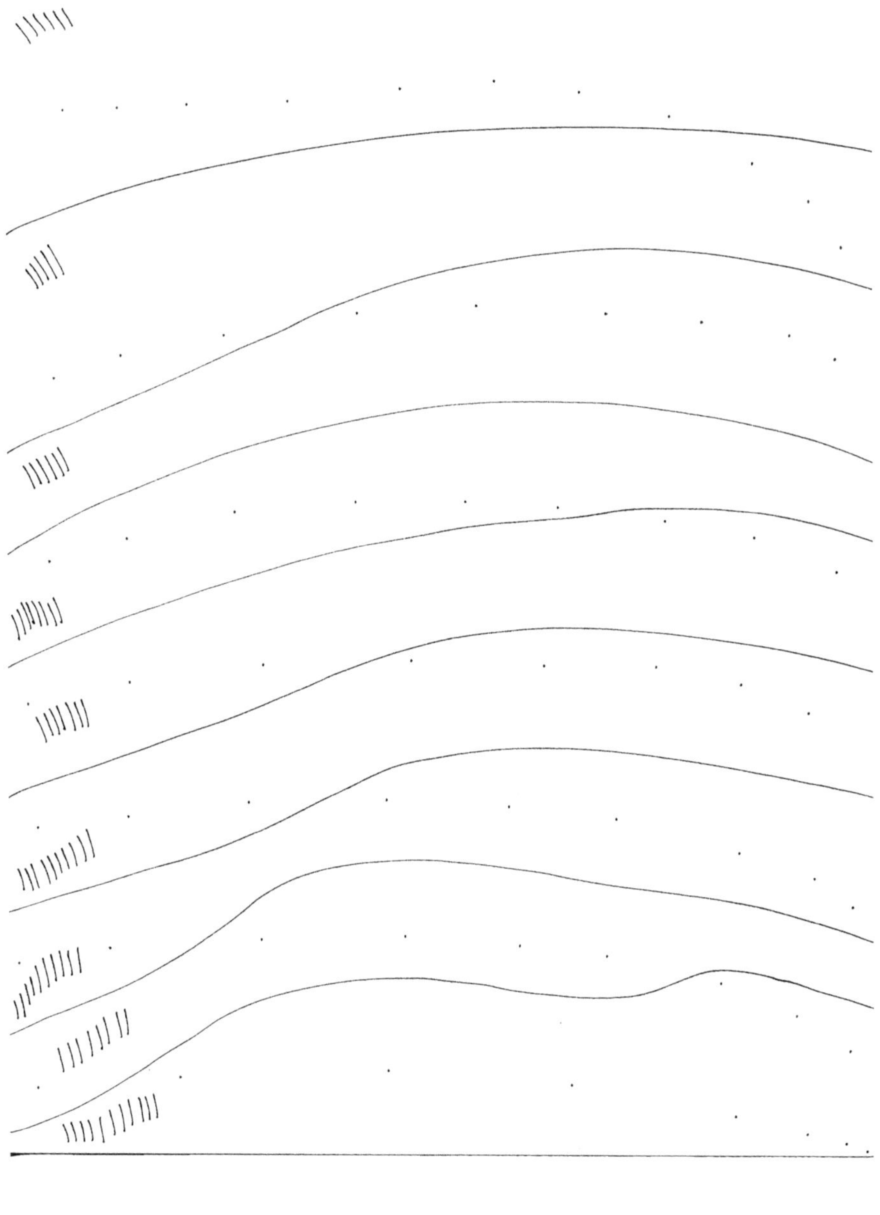

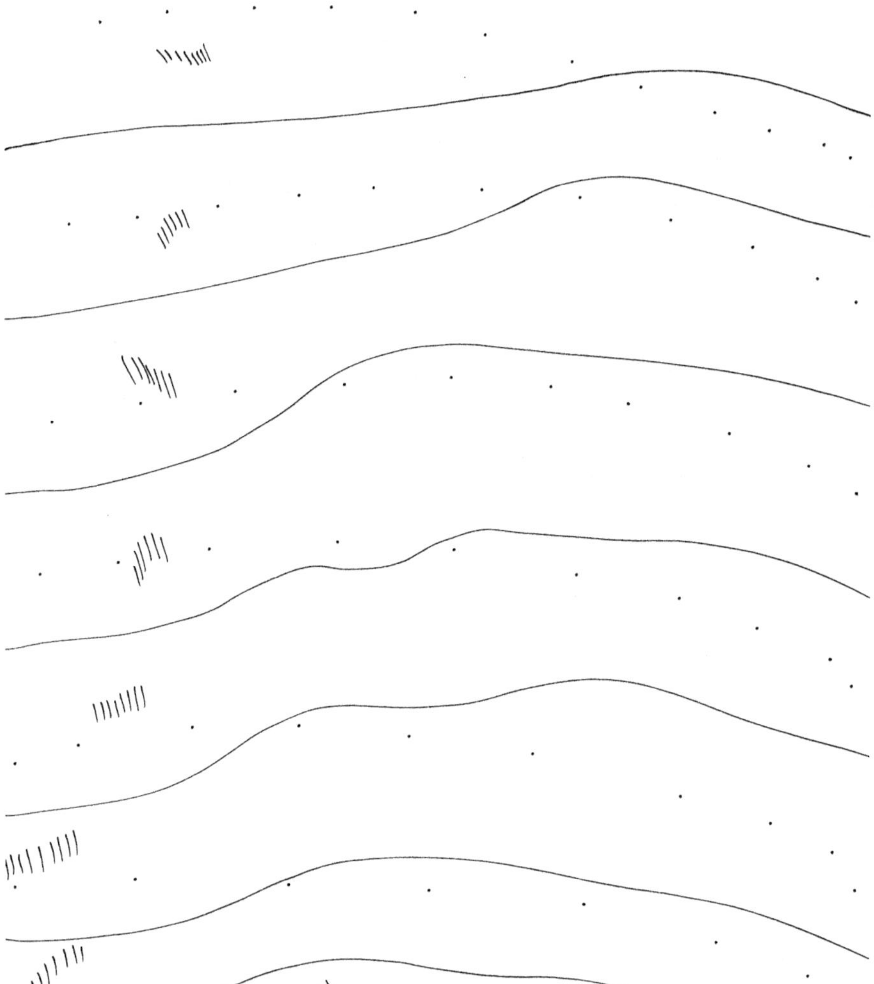

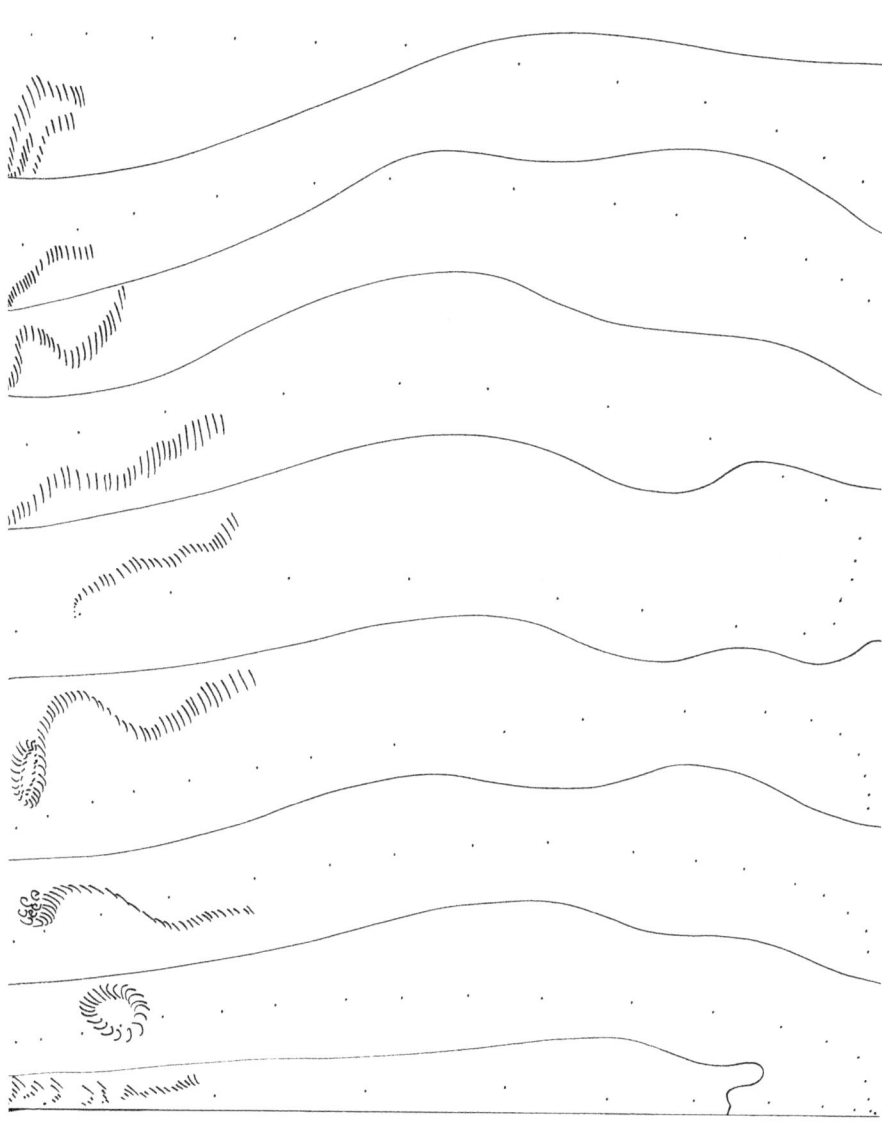

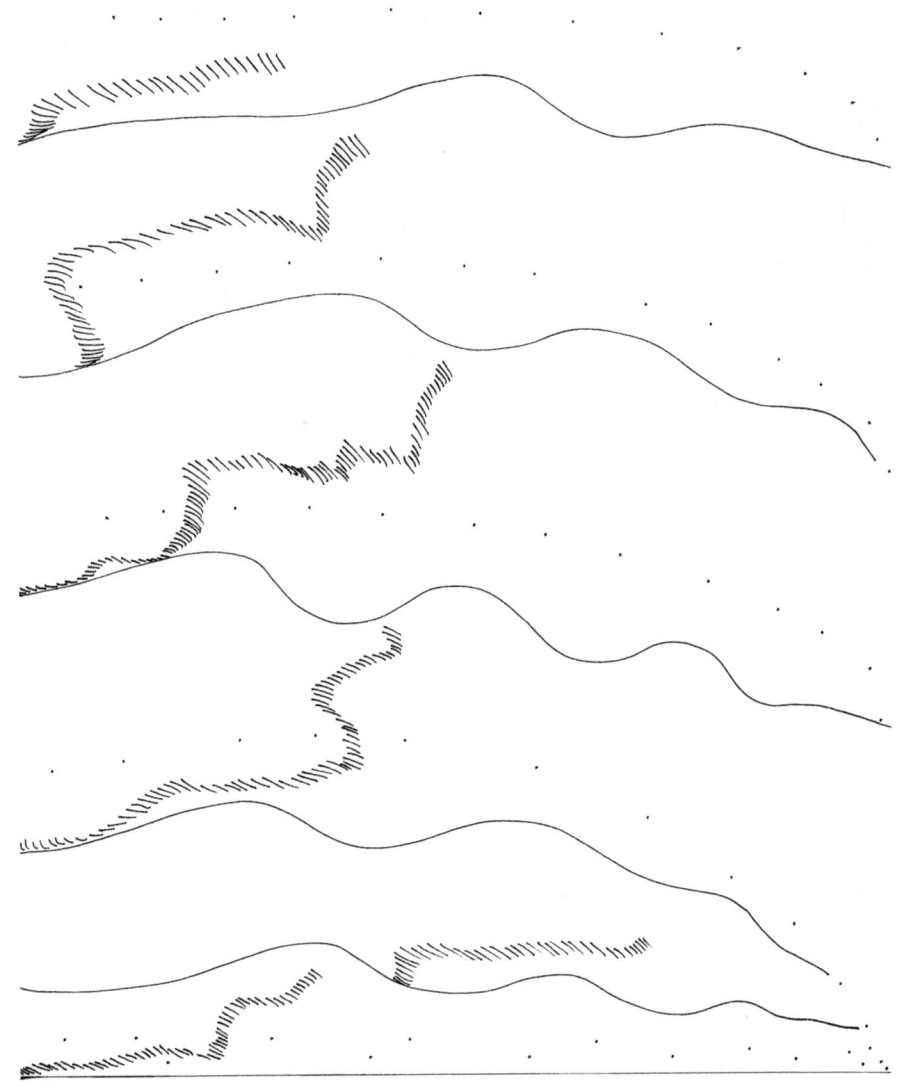

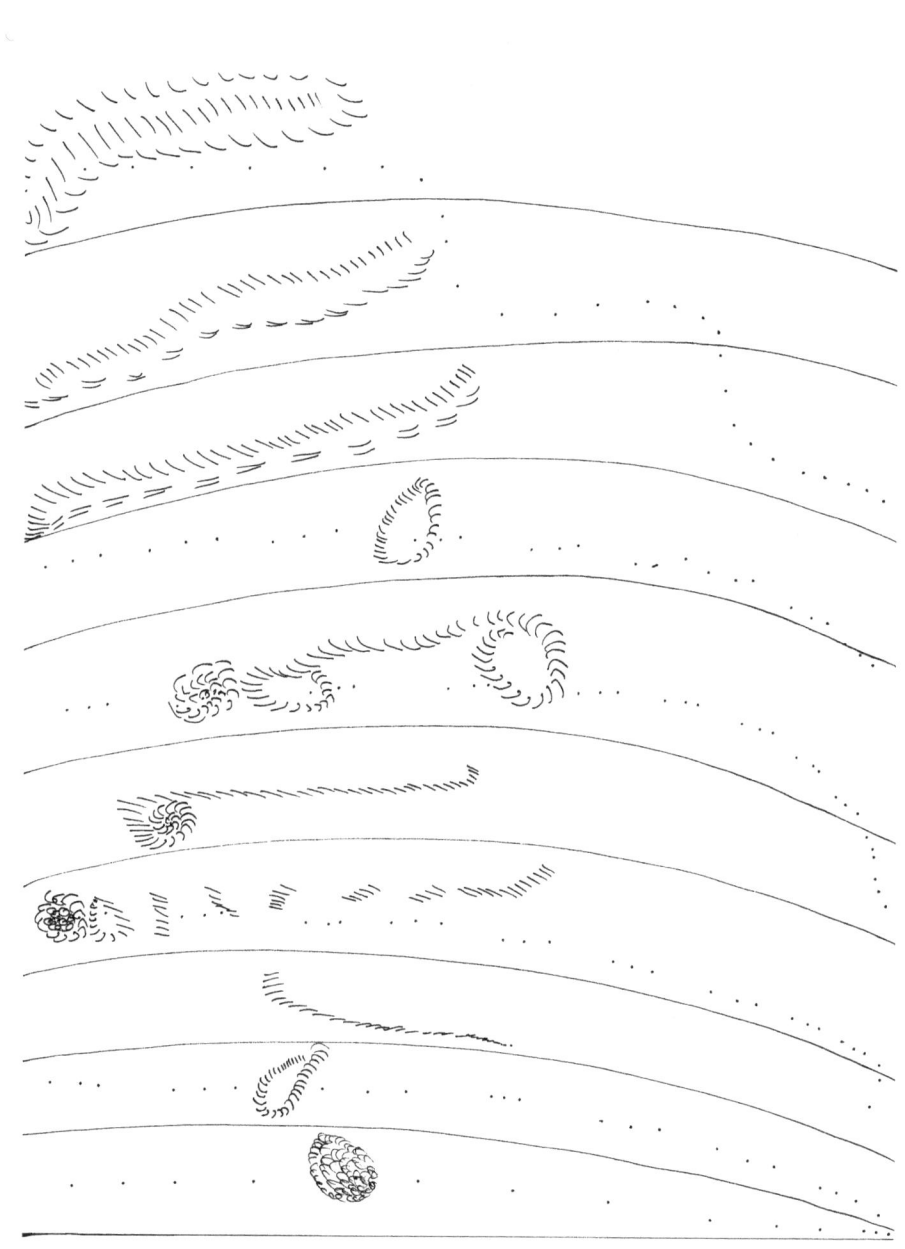

CONTINUED IN VOLUME 2

www.ingramcontent.com/pod-product-compliance
Lightning Source LLC
Chambersburg PA
CBHW080706190526
45169CB00006B/2261